The Feldenkrais® Method is a missing link in lifelong learning. The ability to recognize and feel inborn natural movement patterns becomes the basis for redirecting discomfort and increasing mobility throughout the body—Osa has an ability to share these ideas as they apply to real-life work situations.

Suzanne Hirt, M.Ed., P.T., Professor Emeritus
Physical Therapy Program
Medical College of Virginia
Virginia Commonwealth University

The era of high-speed, high-tech communications has brought to the clinician a patient population that is better informed on health care isssues and much more eager to be both involved with and responsible for their pursuit of wellness than their predecessors. However, patient education by the clinician has traditionally suffered from scheduled time constraints, variable communication skills, and cumbersome manuals with complex illustrations which tend to foster further misunderstanding. In some cases, these formats have been replaced by more simplistic pamphlets in wall racks which may be more confusing than one would hope. The challenge for the professional is to bridge this gulf of fog and miscommunication and provide the informational shortcut to that state of well-being.

Dr. Jackson, in her book, Natural Ease™ for Work, *offers—not a compromise—but a breakthrough in providing useful information which bridges this gulf and enables one to be better informed regarding the wellness concerns which affect their state of being both in leisure and at work. For those who have long suspected that proper posture had something to do with health—regardless of whether you sit in the waiting room or in the clinician's office—this book describes the enjoyable experience that permits the positive physical response and psychological benefit for which you have been searching.*

Timothy E. Eckstein, D.O.
DH Family Practice Center VIII, Inc.
Etna, Ohio

As a friend, colleague and gifted clinician, Osa Jackson-Wyatt has chosen a path of learning. Her excitement about sharing that growth allows you to learn from her experience.

Darcy Umphred, Ph.D., P.T.
Partners in Learning (private practice)
Carmichael, California

Osa brings new perspective in the awareness and recognition of tensions, aches, and pains which are a daily part of life. Her self-help philosophy will help everyone minimize the effects of every-day stresses and increase one's satisfaction with life. This book is excellent reading for those of us who still take personal responsibility for our own well-being.

Peter M. Boruta, M.D.
Rochester Hills Orthopaedics
Rochester, Michigan

Osa communicates clinically relevant concepts with unusual clarity and passion.

She is extraordinarily adept at reaching the heart of her material and her audience. Drawing from a broad range of experience, she is able to share pertinent ideas and practical approaches.

Joan E. Edelstein, Associate Professor
of Clinical Physical Therapy
College of Physicians and Surgeons
Columbia University

Natural Ease™ for Work *is a clear and practical guide integrating awareness with movement. By exploring the simple movement exercises in this book, the reader is able to reprogram their nervous system for better functioning. Certainly, there is a true blending of mind, body, and spirit in helping a person to achieve improvement of daily living.*

Kenneth Fink, D.O.
Farmington, Michigan

We are physicians in practice with a combined experience of forty-five years in taking care of multiple aspects of medicine, including Physical and Rehabilitation Medicine.

Recently we came across a patient self-help book entitled Natural Ease™ for Work by Osa Jackson-Wyatt, Ph.D., P.T., describing different and effective modalities of therapy for pain control and also to prevent or modify musculoskeletal injuries in our daily life. This book deals with important relevance of movement to daily activities of living, increased relaxation and comfort. We are very impressed with the information provided. It is educational, thought-provoking and deals with alternative modalities for improving one's ability to deal with physical strains and stresses of daily life.

I would recommend this book to all my patients and peers without hesitation. It is a great work.

Umesh G. Gowda, M.D.
Rochester Family Physicians, P.C.
Rochester, Michigan

Natural Ease™ for Work

Can You Move to Get
the Job Done?

Printed by Viking Press Inc.
Designed and Composed by Barbara Field
Cover Illustration by Kaethe Zemach-Bersin

Physical Therapy Center
134 W. University, Suite 302
Rochester, Michigan 48307

Printed in the United States of America

Natural Ease™ for Work

Can You Move to Get the Job Done?

Osa Jackson-Wyatt, Ph.D., P.T.

Physical Therapy Center
Rochester, Michigan 48307

*This book is dedicated
to all who are curious
and willing to explore
to find a better way.*

Contents

Illustrations

Acknowledgments

I WANT TO THANK my husband and son for their patience and support. My teachers have helped to shape my vision of lifelong learning. Thank you to Mr. Stelter, Miss Lennon, Mr. Major, Mr. Jenkins, Carola Speads, Moshe Feldenkrais, Hans Selye, Bertha Bobath, Stanley Hoppenfeld, Dr. Cyriax, Dr. Kaltenborn, Traudi Kaltenborn, Olaf Evjenth, and all the students and participants in my courses and workshops. Each person brings a unique perspective to a situation, and I appreciate the kindness and support that has been shown me. The model for the photographs in this book (who is also a wonderful secretary), Lesley Stahl, deserves special mention for her flexibility and patience. As a photographer, I want to acknowledge the dedication to detail given by Rick Smith. My deep gratitude goes to the creative people I work with at the Physical Therapy Center. Working with real people and real clinical problems helps me to learn new insights every day. A special thank you to my parents for all their love and for being role models for lifelong learning.

OSA JACKSON-WYATT, PH.D., P.T.   JULY 1994

How To Use This Book

ANY TASK INVOLVES MOVEMENT, even if it is just the motion of breathing as you sit quietly. As you open this book and look at the pictures and text, let your intuition guide you to what interests you the most. If you feel that starting at the beginning is not for you, then please go to where your interest guides you. If you start reading something that you are curious about, it is likely that you will discover ideas you can use in your life. This follows the old saying, "when the student is ready, the teacher will appear." At some point in the future, go back and try reading the book from beginning to end. Each time you read this book, it can help you discover the state of your "union" (body, mind, and soul). The ability to move and perform the necessary tasks in life reflects your state of being right now. Action and movement involve the union of the body, mind, and soul. The body is only one-third of the formula for action. Movement abilities are an easy way to examine your adaptability. The modification of movement through learning easier ways to move is a way to improve your adaptability. This book presents movement experiments that can help you become aware of your movement abilities and strategies for improving those abilities as long as you live.

Instructions for Learning

LIFE PRESENTS NEW SITUATIONS for you to adapt to every day. Life is an ongoing process of change. Learning to problem solve the situations of life without turning the body into a suit of armored muscular tightness—that is a reasonable goal. This book invites you to evaluate the question: "How much of my Natural Ease™ is locked up by extra muscular tightness?" You may say, "I have never been flexible." Each person inherits basic features in structure (i.e., muscle, bone, tendon). *The game of life is learning how much to tighten to get each job done and then . . . being able to relax and go back to the natural resting length of the muscles that allows an ideal posture for initiating the next new movements for that task.* If you take the time to notice what is most suitable for you, you can prevent or modify many musculoskeletal strains and injuries. Play with the ideas in the book—go slowly and explore what suits you.

The last chapter is provided as a tool for beginning to explore new and more efficient ways to move. The easiest thing to do is to read the last chapter onto an audio tape and then sit down and do the movement lessons. The goal is for you to discover: "What am I ready to learn?" Start with movements that are easy and pain free. If you have any questions about using this book, contact your doctor or a local health care provider trained in the Feldenkrais® Method. A list of qualified professionals by state is available from this address:

Feldenkrais Guild
706 Ellsworth Street
P.O. Box 489
Albany, OR 97321
U.S.A.

Best wishes for lifelong learning!
Osa Jackson-Wyatt, Ph.D., P.T.

Chapter I
Introduction

LIFE IS ABOUT CHANGE. People need to adapt in order to handle the events that occur. Adaptability is the focus of this book, and it is about how to discover the skills needed to enjoy the ongoing demands of real life. Webster says that to adapt is to "make suitable or to make suitable by alteration." Our ease of movement is an outward expression of our ease of adaptation to the day-to-day activities of our lives. Movement or motion is a part of every task or activity that a person needs to use to make life work.

The ability to adapt to the real demands of life involves every aspect of our human self. What kinds of things do people need to learn to adapt to? In every phase of life, there are new skills to master. It starts when we are born, and the need to adapt continues until the end of our lives. As a teenager, life involves learning the ability to sit comfortably for many hours in school, to carry your books, to drive a car, to relax under pressure and take an exam (for the driver's license or college admission test), to speak in front of a group of people, etc. The list of skills required just to be an effective young adult is staggering. Movement and using your body efficiently are a key part of every task mentioned. Now, to top it all off, you master all those skills and graduate from high school, and for about one day, or maybe even one month, you can rest and enjoy the mastery . . . then new challenges appear.

1

You might ask, "How does that apply to me?" As you are learning a new skill, it is easy to become worried or nervous, and the emotions that come with worry can cause you to tighten your body.

How much muscular tightness is needed to get a particular job done? Excitement can bring a little extra tension, just for the moment you walk on stage, and this may help you feel ready. As you actually perform, the Natural Ease™ needs to return for you to perform efficiently. If you get so worried that you tighten your body more than is needed, you will literally begin to be tripped up by the extra tightness.

Early warning signs of extra tightness can include trouble falling asleep at night, needing to take deep breaths often, or a feeling of tightness in your chest. Common early warning signs of extra muscular tightness at rest can be evaluated using the movement experiments included in this book. It was found in formal testing that if a person could not do the movement experiments easily, they were more likely to have a history of difficulties with movement (i.e., pain, limitations in activities, or difficulty finding comfort in basic postures like sitting or standing). The ability to put on appropriate protective tightness and take it off as needed is part of adaptability.

The irony of life is that we each meet unique life experiences that require us to adapt. The first love may come at thirteen, or at the age of thirty-four. The first death in the family may touch you at the age of three or at the age of sixty-three. Life does present challenges. You experience the death of a good friend or relative, you get sick, you get angry, you get overtired, and now the situation requires you to explore emotional skills related to getting along with other people while still taking care of yourself.

On top of a full life that has required ongoing change and adaptability, retirement comes and offers more changes that require more adaptability. The ability to adapt is closely tied to the ability to observe, to notice details, to select new options, and to develop that ongoing urge to improve the situation so it will feel better to you. Notice the word *feel*—it is a word that is personal to each of us. I need to notice what "feels" best for me. I need to make that decision. Can you feel what is best for you? It is a natural process to seek out solutions, activities, and events that feel pleasing and fulfilling to each of us. The long-term results of each person's choice will help reveal if the person was accurate in their self-assessment. The movement experiments presented in this book offer you an opportunity to take inventory of your movement abilities. Doing the movement experiments gives you a chance to notice if your beliefs about your abilities are accurate, realistic, and at the level you feel is needed to do the many jobs/tasks in your daily life.

Adapting to life is a process that is molded and shaped by the uniqueness of who you are. "Who am I?" The way you answer that question is a reflection of what you get excited about, what you enjoy, and what makes you feel safe and comforted. So now the game of life continues. You have chosen to begin to look at yourself for the fun of knowing more about yourself. "Fun?" Many of you will wrinkle your nose, but I insist it is a game of life. Life is to be lived, and if you live it controlling every breath so it is equal and predictable and certain, it will be hard to laugh or to cry. As you come to know yourself better, it will be easier to discover how to adapt to each new challenge that life brings.

Facts of Life

Life involves change and the ability to find enjoyment in the changes. What does this mean? The first step is to admit that there are some aspects of life that cannot be changed. These are the things we need to accept and then make choices about how to work with them. The advantage of accepting things is that you are then free not to worry about them. The following are some examples of aspects of your life that you cannot change:

1. Most of us need to work for a living, and work requires movement (even if it is the task of cleaning your own floor). Even if you do not work to earn money, there is always the

work of taking care of yourself, the place where you live, the people and pets you care about.

2. Some physical abilities, like the ability to run fast for a hundred feet, will be altered somewhat by normal age-related changes.

3. Physical fitness can help you adapt better to the stresses in life.

4. Certain things in life are inevitable, like breathing, death, and taxes. It is also inevitable that, with age, the majority of individuals will find that their metabolism (the speed at which the body burns the fuel/food provided) slows down slightly. This means that unless you increase your activity level (pleasant aerobic exercise—so that your heart increases ten to twenty beats above the resting rate for 10 to 20 minutes a day), you will truly need to eat fewer calories when you are fifty than when you were twenty, or you will gradually become more and more overweight.[1, 2]

5. Improving your muscle strength only helps you to do your job better *if* muscle weakness was the primary cause of your problems.

6. Your effectiveness at work is affected by all of your abilities (mental, emotional, physical, social, and spiritual), your environment and the actual tasks to be done, and your enjoyment or satisfaction in doing the job.

Good News

The good news is that what happened to you in your past does not require you to expect the same activities and outcomes in the future. What does this mean? It means that at any moment in your life, if you have experienced a major loss, the opportunity to grieve is there, and then six months to three years later the adventure of living can proceed again. The ability to dream, to be excited by a project, to be inspired to help another person with a project, all grows out of living in the present, letting yourself be curious and selecting pleasing ways to participate in the life around you. Every human being needs to feel loved and cared about, and to feel needed (i.e., a reason to get up in the morning), and to feel safe and respected with no fear of attack (either verbal or physical).

How Can I Adapt More Effectively?

Learning to adapt can involve many aspects of yourself. Let us begin by describing basic things that can alter movement and your Natural Ease™ at work or play. The foundation concepts for this book are:

1. **PAIN.** When you feel pain, it is presumed that 99 percent of the time it means something is not quite right. Pain means there is a problem—a need to stop and/or a need to try to reorganize. Pain is a signal that something is wrong. Pain can be physical, like when you step on a nail, or when you overwork and the muscles stiffen, or when illness or injury cause major problems in the body. Pain can also come from emotional sources such as when a person "steps on your emotional toes" (hurts your feelings). Pain is a response—a signal to alert you that something is not right. As you perform the movement experiments, it is presumed that if you discover pain (physical or emotional), you will pause and explore ways to decrease the pain or alter its effects in some way. The goal of the movement experiments and the ideas presented here is to have pain be under your control and a tool for you to use to protect yourself from harmful events/things.

   It is presumed that if pain comes at the end of your day, or if pain increases the longer you are doing an activity, what you are doing has something to do with the increase in the pain. Therefore, noticing your pain instead of ignoring it is the first step in your ability to adapt with ease.

2. **SPEED OF ACTIVITY.** It is critical that you do the movements described in this book slowly to avoid causing or increasing pain. The word *slowly* may mean different things to you than it would to your neighbor or to your friends. For the purpose of this discussion, going slowly means that you notice how you would usually perform the task. The speed at which you move in your usual way is called your habitual speed. For these activities, *slowly* means that you go at *half* the speed you usually move, or slower. When you move slower than your usual speed, you are more likely to learn useful information about ways to improve or make the task easier. A slow pace allows more time to notice the details of what you are doing. If the goal is to improve your adaptability, then more detailed information about yourself and your actions will help you make better decisions.

3. **TIGHTNESS OR STIFFNESS IN YOUR BODY.** If you wake up with muscular stiffness in the morning, it may be caused by a variety of physical reasons (overactivity or overusing certain postures during the day, allergies or medical reactions, emotional tension that is expressed by such things as grinding your teeth or clenching your fists in your sleep, etc.). It is important that you explore the possible causes of the muscular pain or stiffness you feel. The first step in solving the pain problem is discovering all the "straws that break the camel's back." The "camel's back," or the area of discomfort for you, is often caused by many factors, with each contributing a small but significant strain. The goal in evaluating all the possible causes of muscular stiffness/pain is to minimize or eliminate those irritants that you have control over (i.e., your mattress, the draft from the window, the table that is too high, or whatever).

4. **EMOTIONS AND MEMORY OF PAIN.** As you explore your abilities to perform the movement experiments presented,

keep in mind that all movement experiments have an emotional component. What does this mean? It means that simply daring to try the experiment (for example, placing your feet flat on the floor and allowing them to rest there) is a choice to participate today and a choice to explore and observe your reactions. After a major injury to your foot, the same experiment that was *easy* before the accident may mean choosing to forget the severe pain that was present six weeks ago. The physical healing may have occurred; the doctor tells you that it is safe and should not cause any major pain. Now the challenge is to trust the information and slowly and gently develop the confidence and the ability to put the weight on your foot *today* and forget the pain from the past. The key is to notice yourself *now*—"Am I tense? "Do I feel muscular tightness and then adjust accordingly?" Another way to say the same thing is that each of us needs time to get used to the novelty of each new situation. Every person needs time to just sit and become aware of the reality of the present moment. "Be present in the here and now!"

5. **FATIGUE.** Learning is easiest when you are well rested. Try to perform the movement experiments when you feel well rested. If you choose to explore/experiment with learning when you are fatigued, it is obviously necessary to go slower and to move with less effort. The rationale for this approach is to provide a margin of ease and safety. (You are more likely to be creative when you are well rested.)

6. **CLOTHING.** You need to be dressed comfortably so that the garments you are wearing do not restrict movements or create areas of irritation or pressure. (Avoid clothes with thick seams like those found in some trousers.) Be sure your slacks or undergarments are not so tight that they leave pressure marks on your body.

7. **THE ENVIRONMENT IN WHICH YOU LEARN.** The place
   you choose to do your learning/reading of this book needs
   to be warm enough that the temperature is not a distracting
   factor. It is well known that if you get too cold, it will distract
   you from monitoring your ease of movement and the details
   of movement. If pets are in the area, they can only help you
   learn if they lay quietly and watch. It may be necessary to go
   into a room alone to do the movement experiments if your
   pets get excited by you getting down on the floor.

8. **MEDICATIONS AND OTHER STIMULANTS.** It is presumed
   that you are taking no medications or drugs that alter your
   sensitivity to monitoring how you feel physically or emotion-
   ally. If you are taking medication that may alter your sensitivity, please discuss using this book with your physician prior
   to proceeding with actually carrying out the movement
   experiments. If you are currently taking medications (pre-
   scription or over-the-counter) that affect your ability to moni-
   tor how you feel, it is likely that the learning activities may
   need to be done more frequently (in order to learn through
   self-exploration) than if you are not using medications.

References

1. Gardner, D.C., Beatty, G.J. *Stop Stress and Aging Now.* New
   Hampshire: American Training and Research Association, Inc.,
   1987.

2. Jackson, Osa (ed). *Physical Therapy and The Geriatric
   Patient,* second edition. New York: Churchill Livingstone Pub.,
   1989.

Chapter II
Know Thyself

Get Moving and Then . . .

ADAPTING IS ABOUT being free to do the things that are important to you. Movement is a part of every action, and one aspect of adapting to events. For example, every day you use one hand more than you use the other. The more "intelligent" hand is the doer of most of your daily activities. What if during your entire lifetime you decided to continue to develop your movement intelligence and abilities? What if you decided to learn to use your "other" hand as much as you do the one that is your dominant hand? The capacity of the brain to learn to be more ambidextrous (using the right hand and the left hand with nearly equal ability) can be helpful for adults of any age.

What Are You Saving Your Brain For?

The ability to use both hands easily can minimize strain and actually prevent overuse injuries (i.e., when the right hand is tired, switch the tool to the left hand). Another major advantage of learning to move with ease and coordination with the nondominant hand is that it will help prevent overuse tightness in such areas of your body as the neck, shoulders, and rib cage, as well as the lower back. The freedom to switch when fatigued can allow someone to work longer on a project they are excited about and with greater ease. Adapting to life involves the ability to keep learning new skills. If this idea is taken to the extreme, *it means that you can learn to become more coordinated and creative as long as you live.*

Now ask yourself a question. Compared to ten years ago, are you enjoying running or jumping less, or do you notice less ease of movement even in walking to do your shopping? If you answer yes, in most cases these changes are *not* related to normal aging. If there is no injury or illness, it is possible that the changes are related to accumulated protective tightness, work-related repetitive overuse tightness, and/or a decrease in overall physical fitness, or any combination of these causes.

You are invited to observe how you automatically (without thinking about it) organize your body for the basic life activities. The sample task will be to learn to do something with your nondominant hand.* You may usually perform the task with your right hand, but now you will begin to experiment to learn how to do the task easily with your left hand, or vice versa. For example, what if you begin with easy and safe activities and switch from using your dominant hand to performing the task using your nondominant hand? What kinds of activities could you do? What about a game of Ping-Pong with your nondominant hand, or brushing your teeth with your nondominant hand? Switching the hand you use for easy activities will allow automatic changes in your body that will soften and make the resting tension of your muscles closer to what is ideal or "normal." But this is only true if the activity is pleasant and feels easy for you. At first, this means that you need to do the activity gently so it really "feels" pleasant to you. Also, it is easier to learn and improve the ability to move if you feel that there is plenty of time. Don't rush.

Extra tension at rest. When you move, or when you sit and rest, the skeleton (your bones) can provide the major structural sup-

---

* Your dominant hand is the one you prefer to write with and perform most self-care tasks (brushing your teeth or combing your hair).

port. The muscles are meant to be at rest when you relax (i.e., sit quietly) and then to tighten (contract) to perform an action. If one action or posture is used too much, the muscles may lose their ability to "park," meaning the ability to relax (no effort when at rest). Overused areas or muscle groups will tend to have the muscles more tight at rest than is desirable. This will make the area increasingly tender to the touch (trigger points), and perhaps uncomfortable (awkward, feeling tense, unable to find a restful, easy position), and the posture may feel undependable. When you try to move the tight muscles, they will create a motion that may feel uncoordinated. Another example is that moving the ankle requires a particular pattern of action that primarily involves the muscles of the lower leg and foot. If you are anxious, then as you try to move your ankle you may also tighten your hip, clench your jaw, and hold your breath. The simple ankle motion (moving your foot) has become a very overpriced effort involving many parts of the body with no direct improvement in the ankle motion. The ankle motion that should cost $5 worth of energy now costs you $50 worth of energy. The emotions of worry and fear can make you alter your movements and you become very inefficient in your ability to adapt.

Extra tension in action. It is my observation that a higher than desirable resting tension in any part of the body over long periods of time can make a person more prone to accidents and falling. The ultimate problem is that a muscle or muscle group that is tighter than necessary at rest is less adaptable, and those muscles will ultimately make the owner (you) feel more awkward/not as coordinated and less likely to enjoy physical activities. One of the worst results is that the rigidity or tightness in the body can make you say, "I can't sleep anywhere except in my own bed." So . . . no more vacations? No more visits to friends? Family? The good news is that in the majority of cases, the individual can learn to relax again and become more adaptable. Enjoying life requires ongoing adaptability and the ability to problem solve to discover and gradually eliminate any extra tension at rest or in action.

Aging . . . Me? What Does It Mean?

Now you say, "I am ____ years old. I can't expect to be adaptable at my age." Whether you are forty, seventy, or ninety, adaptability is more a state of mind than a condition of the body. Norman Vincent Peale, Rose Kennedy, George Burns—these well-known people have been passionately involved in making their unique contributions to life well into their later years. My response to you is that as you dare to know yourself better, you can explore, learn, and adapt to the demands of life and passionately pursue your own dreams. The example I like to use is that of a driver sitting in a car with the side windows blackened. If you do not know what is to the right and to the left of you, it is likely you will be less effective as a driver on the highway of life. Similarly, the more you know about yourself, how you move, what you can do to make reaching or lifting easier, the safer and simpler it will be for you to do basic tasks (i.e., turn your head to see to back up your car) or to work toward your goals.

As you contemplate doing the basic flexibility experiments in this book, think about the last time you had a thorough physical examination by your doctor. If you are over the age of thirty, and if it has been two years since your last physical, please consider having a physical prior to reading further. Why? An ounce of prevention is worth a pound of cure (a famous person said that). You say, "I don't have time." Or, "I feel great." I would reply that a physical is your responsibility as part of preventing unnecessary illness or injury. It is your doctor's job to take good care of you when you get sick. It is your responsibility as an adult to be aware of the obvious health maintenance activities (i.e., getting enough rest, flossing and brushing your teeth). Today science has demonstrated many ways to improve health. *It is your job to participate in your health care.* Are you taking reasonably good care of yourself and living in the twentieth century? For example, it is a well-known fact that breast self-examination and other screenings have improved the recovery rate for women after breast cancer. Another advantage of preventive health care is that if you get sick, the doctor knows what you looked like and how you acted when you were feeling good. "So what?" you ask.

1. By visiting your doctor for a physical, you can be sure that you and your doctor get along. If you don't like your doctor when you feel good, how are you going to get along in a crisis or illness situation?

2. If you go for periodic checkups, the doctor gets to know you and your family and will be able to take into account all the emotional/spiritual/social factors that can play into your recovery. The doctor who has known you for years can also know your uniqueness.

"So what?" you ask again. Well, I will tell you my story. My resting blood pressure is about 102/60, and, yes, I feel great. The textbook says that 120/80 is average. We know that I am not average. None of us is average in every aspect of ourselves. I got sick, and in two days my blood pressure rose to 139/80 at rest. I had sensations of pressure in my eyes and a headache, and I went to my doctor. I was lucky he recognized that something was drastically wrong because he knew my previous blood pressure and because I myself insisted that he look at the fact that the change occurred so quickly; also, I could report what was my "healthy, normal blood pressure," and I got the care I needed. If my doctor had not known me, or if I had not been medically trained, or if my doctor had chosen not to listen to my interpretation of what was normal for me, there is less likelihood that he would have known what to do to help me get better. (The increase in blood pressure was a complication during my pregnancy that was successfully treated, and I had a healthy 10-pound baby boy!)

Now it is your turn to get into action. For the average person, the movement experiments in this book can seem very easy. If these motions feel natural—congratulations. If at any point as you do the movements you feel pain, do less or stop. You can alter the speed of motion, the position, and/or how you breathe. The key is to keep the movements *feeling easy*. Your goal is to discover who you are today. As you learn how much is easy for you to do today, then you can slowly work to improve in the tasks you feel are important to you. I salute your uniqueness and I encourage you to take good care of yourself. Good luck on your journey of discovery to find the new movement skills needed for lifelong learning and adapting to accomplish your desired goals.

Chapter III
How Do I Move?

OUR EASE OF MOVEMENT is an outward expression of our ease of adaptation to the day-to-day demands of our lives.* Movement can be felt and it can be seen. Although I may wish to know about my ease of adapting to an activity, I can lie to myself with words; I can even force myself to believe the lies. Today, however, technology exists that does not allow you to lie about movement. A motion done three times in a row can be recorded to show your unique habitual movement pattern.

The movements included for your personal evaluation are among the basic movements commonly used in day-to-day activities. For each movement you are to perform, the possible results of doing the experiment will be described. Directions will be given on how to move and how to carry out the movement experiment. The common ways that people "cheat," or substitute by using other parts of their body, or how people might adapt if they do it very quickly with a strong effort, will also be discussed. Lastly, helpful hints will be given so you can explore ways to make the movements easier. Sample tasks in which each basic movement ability is needed in

*It is presumed that you feel good and have no acute illness. If you currently have a fever or severe pain, wait to actually do the movements. An option is to think through the movements and practice mentally if that feels pleasant.

daily life will be presented as the rationale for you to include this ability in your repertoire if it is not already there.

If a new position or activity causes mild pain, pulling, or discomfort, stop, rest, and try again after you are free of pain.

Do not cause yourself discomfort. Flexibility screening using the movement experiments listed below can be done in any order. It is recommended that you work through the experiments with a friend. The definition of a "friend" is someone who cares about you and highlights your strengths and does not dwell on your underdeveloped abilities (movements that you cannot perform efficiently). As you work together, you can share the learning and support each other in choosing to adapt in new and more effective ways to perform the job or desired task.

Movement Experiments

Note: You are reminded to work at a comfortable level of exertion or effort. Do not cause even mild discomfort. If you cause pain, you are less likely to enjoy movement/physical activities. The goal is to identify what is pain-free and easy and then work safely from that point toward further improvement in abilities. Use the score sheet beginning on page 88 of this chapter to rate yourself for each movement experiment.

1. Sitting

FUNCTIONAL QUESTION:

1a. Can you sit with ease without a backrest for 3 to 5 minutes? (Use the "Rate Yourself" score sheet.)

Rate yourself: 1. feels natural; 2. can do but with effort; 3. can do but irritates; 4. can do but causes pain; 5. cannot do/choose not to do.

Common signs of trying too hard, overuse, or fatigue: When you sit, you may place your feet behind your knees instead of resting them flat on the floor, and your heels may be lifted off the floor (see Figure 1). Your chest may be rounded, as if sunk down toward your stomach (see Figure 2). There may be no contact on your sitting bones (the two bones in your buttocks meant for sitting on). Your head may be forward (see Figure 3). All these postural disturbances require that the muscles on the front of the body be tighter at rest than is usual or ideal. To sit with ease, the bones of the skeleton need to align properly to help support your body weight in an efficient way (see Figure 4).

Hints to improve Natural Ease™: The various suggestions for increasing the ease of sitting need to be tried one at a time. If any suggestion to improve sitting is not easy and causes pain, stop and rest. If you discover that many of the suggestions are not easy for you, contact your physician/physical therapist for advice.

A comfortable chair to sit on is a major help in sitting with physical ease. The dimensions of your chair need to be suited to your unique body shape (see Figures 5a and 5b). This means that a person who is 4′9″ tall needs a different chair with different dimensions to sit comfortably than a person who is 5′10″. The dilemma in our culture is that the average dining room set is designed for the person who, until 40 years ago, was likely to pay for the dining room set. The average dining room table suits the dimensions of a person who is approximately 5′10″ tall.

If we want to increase physical ease for sitting, then:

1. The chair needs to have a flat, comfortable seat and be the same height in the front as in the back of the seat or be inclined down toward the front of the chair.

2. When you sit on the chair, your feet need to rest flat on a stable, strong surface (the floor or a footstool). The feet need to be the same width apart as your hips so the legs can rest naturally apart (see Figure 6).

It is desirable that when you sit, your thighs are parallel to the floor. What does that mean? Take a round object, like a

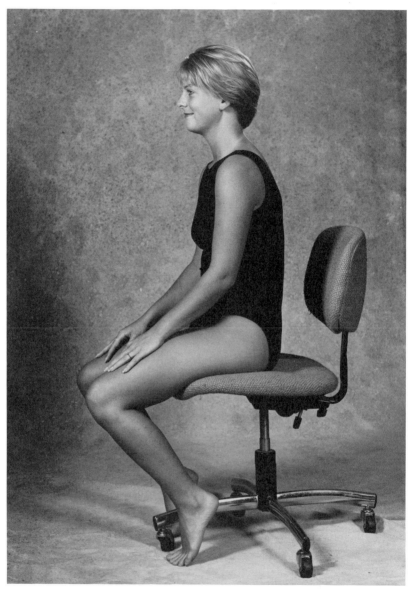

Figure 1. Trying to find comfort by placing feet behind knees—
avoid if possible.

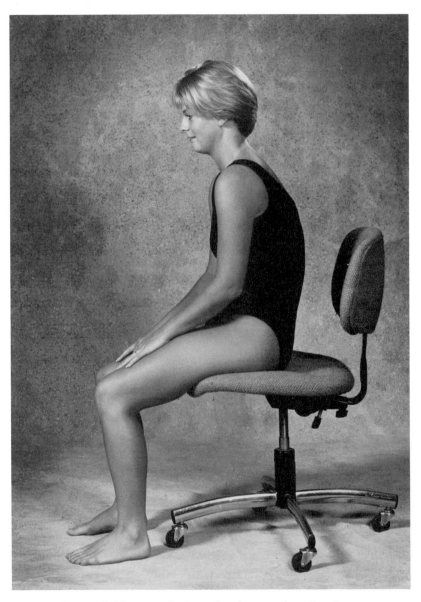

Figure 2. Trying to find comfort by rounding the chest.

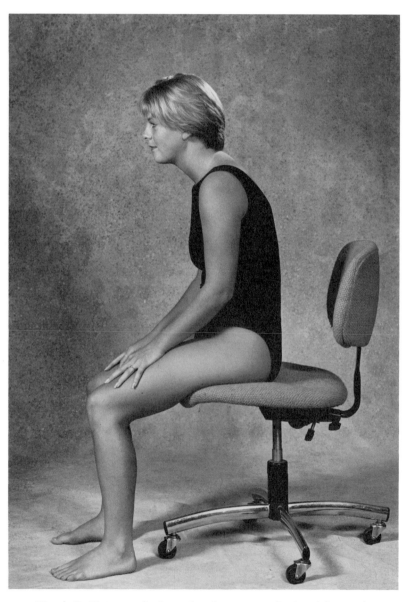

Figure 3. Trying to find comfort by moving the head forward.

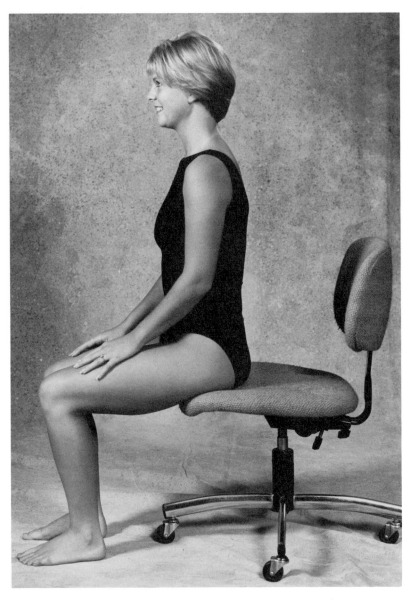

Figure 4. Sitting with head above shoulders and feet
under knees.

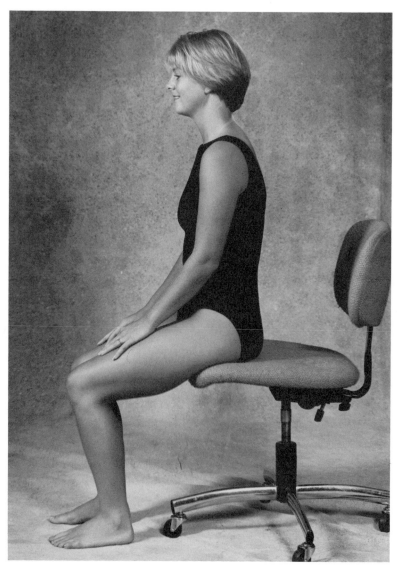

Figure 5a. Chair is too tall.

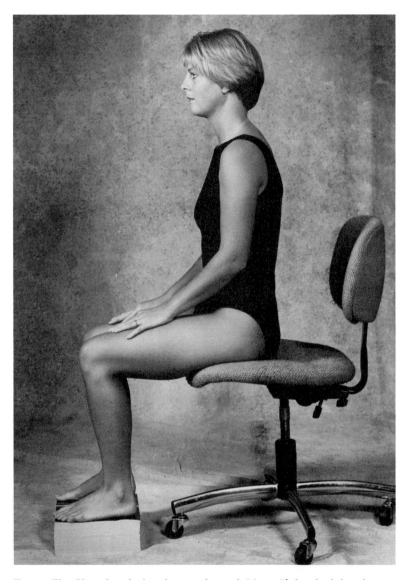

Figure 5b. Chair height has been adjusted. Note: If the desk height can be lowered, it is simpler to do that than to raise the chair. If the desk height cannot be lowered and the chair height is raised, a footstool (i.e., telephone books) can help improve sitting comfort.

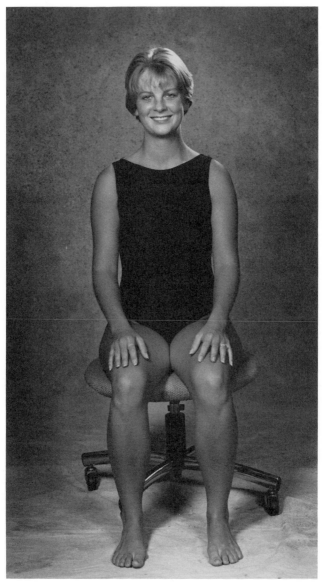

Figure 6. Front view of legs resting with feet flat at the natural hip width apart.

pencil, and place it on your thigh, halfway between your knees and your hips. If the pencil rolls down toward your knees, the chair is too high for you (see Figure 7). This means that you need a tall footstool or other object that will raise your feet. If the pen rolls toward your hips, the chair is too low (see Figure 8). This means that you will need to raise the height of the chair seat.

3. To raise the height of the chair seat to suit you, place a pad or folded towel on the seat of the chair until the pen rests without moving on the middle of your thigh. You are now sitting in a chair that is customized to your height and the length of your legs, and there is a real chance for comfort and ease in sitting (see Figure 9). You can easily make a permanent pad or cushion that you can carry in a briefcase so that you "bring your sitting comfort with you."

4. The backrest for the chair needs to be adjustable to provide a curved support where your lower back arches naturally (see Figure 10). If you have a standard chair, this means that you can use a towel roll (put tape around it to hold it in the desired shape) or a small pillow to provide the back support (if the chair is not suited to your body dimensions). The goal is to allow a slight natural curve in the lower back (lumbar spine—from just above the belt line and down 2 inches or more in the average person) so that the skeleton can help support the body while sitting (see Figure 11).

NOTE: IMPORTANT IDEAS

1. Do not suck in your stomach when sitting—this is an old wives' tale. Pulling in your stomach while you are sitting creates an unnatural strain on your lower back and disturbs your natural lower back posture. At rest, your lower back arch and your belly create a natural balance so that the skeleton can do most of the work of holding you upright while sitting.

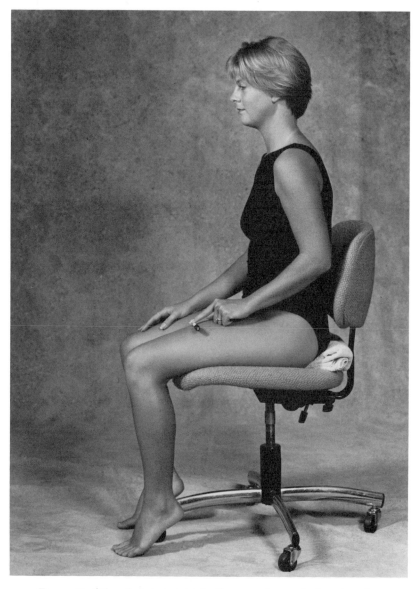

Figure 7. If the chair is too high, the round pencil placed in the
middle of your thigh will roll toward
your knees when you let it go.

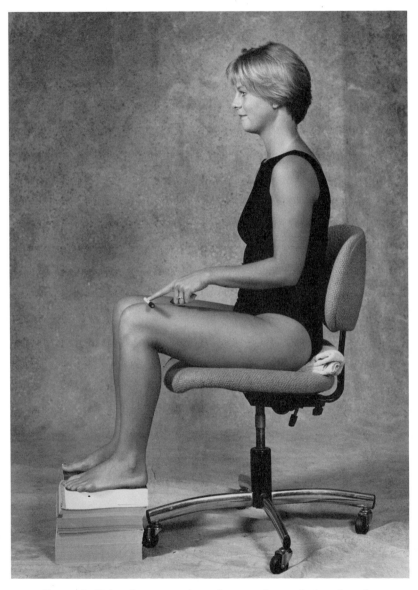

Figure 8. If the chair is too low, the round pencil placed in the
middle of your thigh will roll toward
your hips when you let it go.

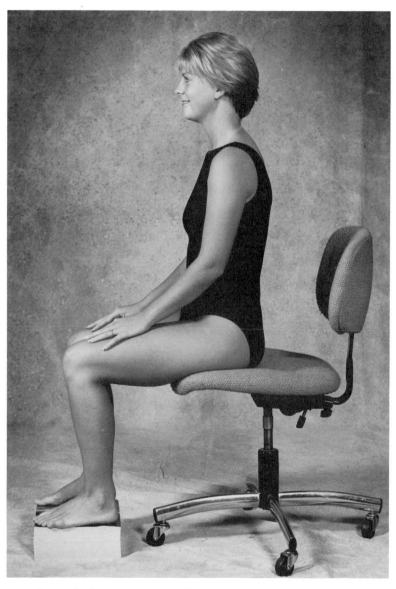

Figure 9. Sitting with chair height adjusted so legs can relax at rest (thighs parallel to floor).

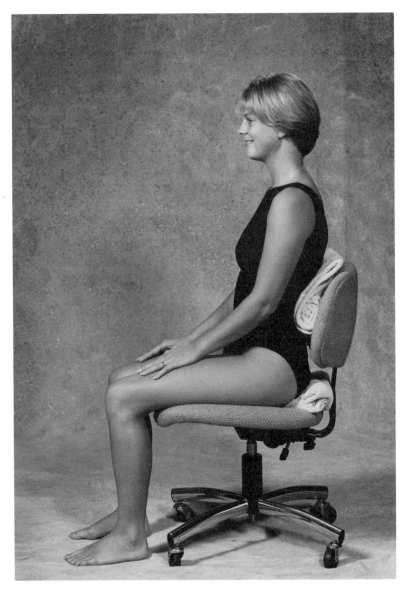

Figure 10. Chair seat raised in back so that seat is level (same
height at front and back of seat). Towel roll is placed
at waistline as a lumbar roll customized to size of body.

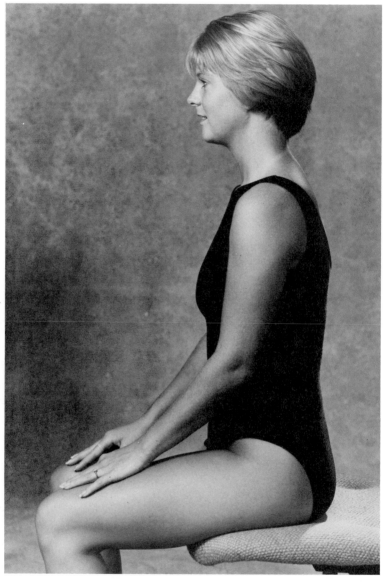

Figure 11. Lumbar curve is meant to be a curve that starts
near the waistline (below elbow level when
shoulders and arms hang naturally).

2. The depth of the chair needs to allow your back to touch the backrest and at least two fingers' width of space between the back of your legs and the front edge of the chair (see Figure 12).

FUNCTIONAL QUESTION:

1b. Is sitting in a neutral pelvic tilt comfortable? (Use the "Rate Yourself" score sheet.)

Rate yourself: 1. feels natural; 2. can do but with effort; 3. can do but irritates; 4. can do but causes pain; 5. cannot do/choose not to do.

A "neutral pelvic tilt," what is that? A neutral pelvic tilt means that you can arch your lower back slightly without any major effort and your buttocks are further back on the chair than the edge of your waistband or belt (see Figure 13). The arch of the lower back lets the skeleton do its natural work of supporting you. Try a small experiment. If you curve your spine/round your back at the waist and below, and literally slouch and let yourself roll back toward the back of the chair, you will feel how your upper body will also round and your head will move forward (see Figure 14).

With a neutral pelvic tilt, the lower part of the body, including the sitting bones, is stacked in a way that the skeleton is most efficient in helping you sit. This means that the two sitting bones (the hard bones in your buttocks that you sit on) need to be used on a daily basis for sitting. As you slouch and use the fleshier part of yourself, your upper body rounds and the advantage (mechanical/coordination) of the pelvic tilt to support your upper back is decreased or totally lost.

Using a pelvic tilt posture is the basis for movement and power in sitting and standing because the largest muscles of the body are attached to the lower body. If you choose not to rest the pelvis/lower body in the ideal resting position, then as you try to move, there is no dependable and mechanically sound base for

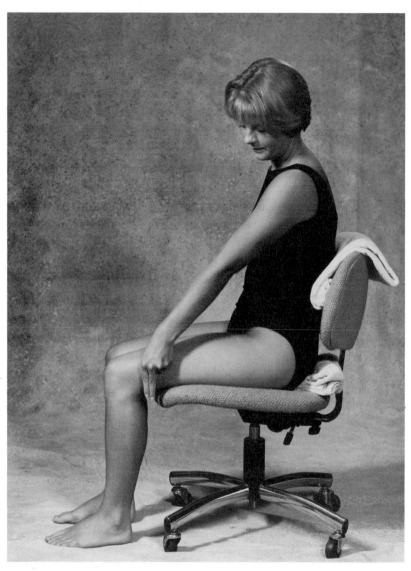

Figure 12. The depth of the chair (distance from front edge of seat to back edge) should allow at least the width of two fingers between upper calf and edge of chair. Note: If chair is too deep, add prop to backrest.

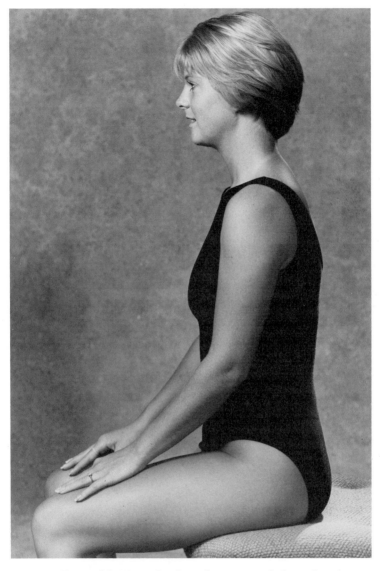

Figure 13. Neutral pelvic tilt means a slight arch
(without any major effort) of the lumbar spine and
your buttocks farther back on chair than
your waistband/belt.

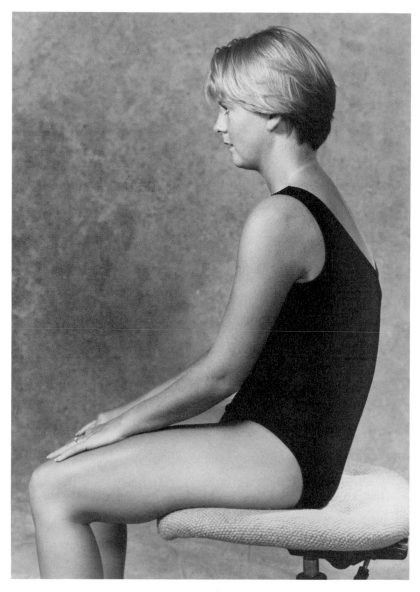

Figure 14. Slouching occurs when there is no neutral pelvic tilt and head moves forward.

beginning the desired motion. Not using a neutral pelvic tilt (not sitting on your sit bones and using that small natural arch in the lower back on a daily basis) increases the likelihood that you will feel less comfortable as you try to sit for longer periods of time.

You might say, "It doesn't feel easy to sit up straight—I have an urge to slouch."

What causes you to slouch and not use what is a natural sitting posture? One common problem is that the furniture does not encourage you to sit with Natural Ease™ (chair is too tall or too short). Another common reason for slouching relates to how you may feel emotionally/spiritually or socially.

If you feel in control, if you feel you can handle the situations that you are asked to participate in, then you are more likely to sit on your sitting bones. If you feel too tall, then you may not choose to act from that base of support by sitting in a posture that is reasonable and organized. If you find that sitting in a natural, upright posture, as shown in Figure 13, is not easy or comfortable for you, it may be due to physical reasons, the furniture, and/or your feelings. As you learn to regain the ability to sit on your sitting bones, there will be changes and new learning related to both how you approach a situation and how you use your physical body in that situation.

FUNCTIONAL QUESTION:

1c. Hip hinge—can you lean forward bending only at hips and pelvic area? (Use the "Rate Yourself" score sheet.)

Rate yourself: 1. feels natural; 2. can do but with effort; 3. can do but irritates; 4. can do but causes pain; 5. cannot do/choose not to do.

When sitting on a chair, lean forward moving only at the hips and pelvic area (do not bend your lower back). Keep your knees at a natural (hip width) distance apart (see Figure 6). This will allow the muscles of the entire lower body to rest on the skeleton in an organized way. In many cultures, sitting like this is discouraged for women. This is also an old wives' tale. If women want to deliver babies with greater ease and be able to control their ability to urinate in a normal fashion when they get to be sixty or seventy years old, they need to be encouraged to use a natural sitting posture that maintains the healthy movements of a normal "pelvic floor." What is that? The pelvic floor is the bottom of the trunk of the body, and it is held together by a series of muscles suspended from the bones in the pelvis and the back. This entire group of muscles is involved in bathroom and sexual activity. So if you wish to have normal bathroom and sexual ease and well-being, then sitting in a natural, easy position is helpful.

"Oh no, I love to sit with my legs crossed," you say. That is okay—the urge to cross your legs, I believe, is like the urge to scratch your nose. Go ahead and cross your legs, just like you might scratch your nose. *Enjoy* crossing your legs—lean forward bending only at the hips (called a hip hinge movement), enjoy the ease and gentle stretching you may feel, and then just as you put your hand down after you scratch your nose, uncross your legs and sit with Natural Ease™. You will be sitting on your sitting bones and resting in a natural way with a functional pelvic floor posture. So, starting in a comfortable sitting position (see Figure 15), bend forward moving only at the hips and pelvic area (see Figure 16).

At rest, your feet need to be below your knees and flat on the floor (see Figure 17). Think of your feet as the foundation that supports your legs in sitting, along with your sitting bones. If your feet are not flat on the floor, then your skeleton cannot do its job and your muscles begin to increase in tension while sitting at rest. An equally important reason is that you are reinforcing natural movement patterns by the positions in which you choose to rest a part of your body. As a therapist, I have observed that it seems easier for people to recover their footing when they slip if they choose to sit in a natural flat-footed posture (with their feet flat on the ground most of the time) as they rest. The theory is that by sitting in a balanced posture you reinforce the habit of useful alignment in your ankles

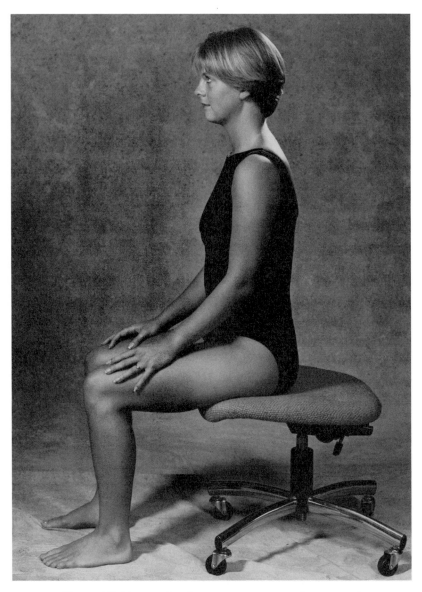

Figure 15. To start hip hinge motion, sit with a neutral
pelvic tilt.

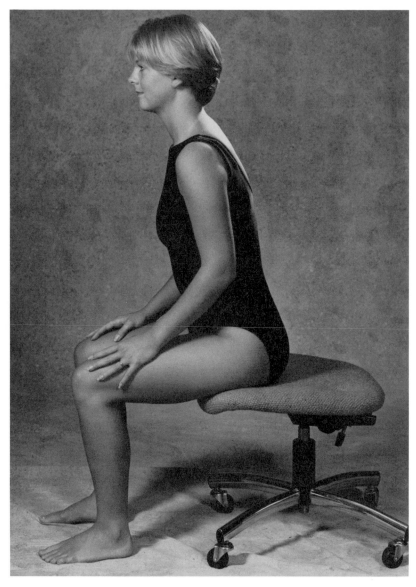

Figure 16. Lean entire trunk (head and spine) forward with motion
occurring *only* at the hips and pelvic area.

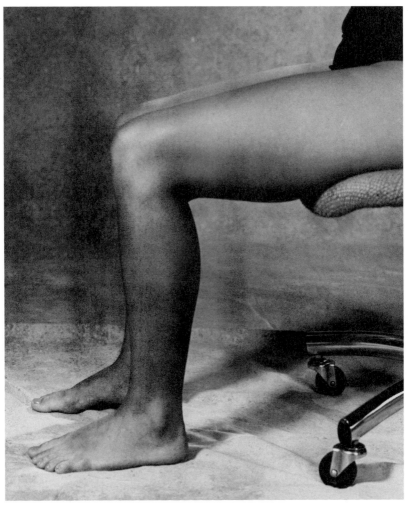

Figure 17. Efficient resting position with feet below knees.

and feet. As you slip and begin to fall, your brain will call forth your ability to bring yourself upright. Your brain will use the ankle action patterns that are habitual and most common, and if you habitually (usually) sit with your feet flat, it appears to be easier to organize those motions to create a safe landing for yourself. Relax as needed, but try to use a flat-footed resting posture most of the time.

NOTE: Move and read as needed and take breaks as you read. Think of them as commercial breaks. If you don't get up every 10 to 20 minutes, or at least stop and stretch, it is easy for your sitting to interfere with your Natural Ease™. Changing positions periodically is another way to promote the Natural Ease™ of movement and overall well-being. An example of a change in position is to lean the majority of your weight to one side and then bring yourself back to sitting evenly.

Hints to improve Natural Ease™: In sitting, the arms should rest comfortably in the lap, and the neck and shoulders need to be at ease. If the position of placing your arms at rest on your lap does not allow your shoulders to relax, then place a pillow on your lap and lay your arms on top. Let your elbows hang with ease *directly below* your shoulders. If this is not comfortable, use a second pillow and notice if that begins to make you feel more comfortable (see Figure 18). *You are responsible for noticing how you feel.* Some individuals may need up to four pillows so that their arms are resting almost at shoulder level before the neck begins to feel at ease and able to relax. This can mean that there is a great deal of tightness present in the neck, shoulders, and/or chest. If you need more than two pillows to allow your neck and shoulders to feel comfortable with your arms resting in your lap, please contact your physician or physical therapist, as this may be a sign that some intervention is needed to prevent further problems.

To increase relaxation for driving, adjusting the angle of the steering wheel, the height of the seat, and the distance of the seat from the steering wheel can promote ease in the shoulders/neck and

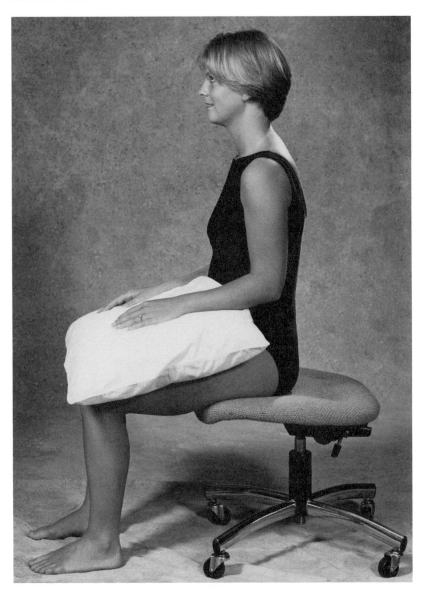

Figure 18. Let elbows hang directly below shoulders to enhance
Natural Ease™. Note: Add one or more pillows
to increase shoulder/neck comfort.

back. The goal is to position yourself so that your elbows are below your shoulders in a comfortable way.

Another experiment you can try is simply to notice the position of your hands. Some people will rest their hands in their lap by literally putting their hands between their legs and resting them on the surface of the chair. Some people will put their hands flat on their thighs, some will put the back of their hands on their thighs with the palms up, some will cross their arms on their chest, and some will feel most comfortable if their arms are hanging at their sides and not in their lap. Try each of the positions mentioned and note which one is most comfortable for you. Rest your arms in the position that feels easiest for you.

In terms of adaptability, the ideal situation is to develop (over your lifetime) the ability to easily use any of these hand positions for daily activity for short periods of time. If you are able to sit with your arms, legs, or any part of your body in a variety of positions, it will increase your overall adaptability.

While you sit, your face needs to be at rest and your jaw needs to be relaxed with your teeth not touching and your tongue resting comfortably. Your eyes can be either open or closed. Use the eye position that is most reasonable for you. If you find that not having your teeth touching creates an awkwardness or a sense of irritation and pressure in your face, then assume a posture with your jaw and teeth that is comfortable for you. As you sit, there will be less strain on your jaw area if your teeth are not constantly forced to touch. If you tend to clench your jaw and rest with your teeth touching, stop and relax your mouth. Ask yourself, "Why am I holding my jaw tight?" Answering this question involves exploring your reactions— "When do I clench my jaw the most? When do I do this the least?" If you have any special pulling, pressure, or pain in the jaw area, contact your physician or physical therapist for advice.

Relevance of movement to daily living: Sitting is a basic posture for social activities and is used in many tasks where the work involves using one or both of the arms and/or the legs. Sitting may be required for work, and taking breaks from sitting as you fatigue is critical to Natural Ease™ and well-being. Sitting is also a posture you need if you spend time behind the wheel of a car or truck. When sitting is not efficient, all arm/leg activities performed when sitting will gradually become strenuous and uncoordinated. What does this mean? If you do not begin to find a more efficient way to sit, eventually pain or other difficulties can develop in the chest, the neck, the shoulders, etc. Sitting in a poor position causes the muscles in the trunk (the neck, chest, and lower back) to function in a rigid manner (bonelike) and not allow the natural movement that promotes normal circulation and normal coordination of the muscles.

2. Pushing Using Your Hands, Arms, and Shoulders

FUNCTIONAL QUESTION: Can you *push your palms together* with the entire palm, fingertips, and fingers touching and your forearms in a straight line and hold for 30 seconds? (See Figure 19.) (Use the "Rate Yourself" score sheet.)

Rate yourself: 1. feels natural; 2. can do but with effort; 3. can do but irritates; 4. can do but causes pain; 5. cannot do/choose not to do.

Common signs of trying too hard, overuse, or fatigue: Hiking up your shoulders toward your ears, elevating your elbows, and/or clenching your teeth together.

Hints to improve Natural Ease™: Check that you are sitting in the easy sitting posture described previously with support for the back as needed. Allow your entire focus to be on whether your palms and fingers touch in a natural, comfortable way. Slowly push your palms together so you increase the pressure. Avoid working so hard that you hold your breath. Breathing is a natural life-sustaining function. This experiment is not a life or death activity, and holding your breath only means that you are taking all of this too seriously.

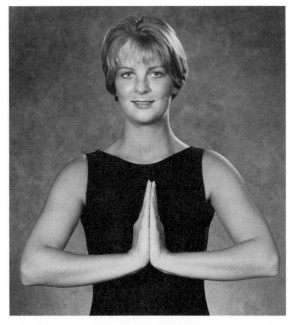

Figure 19. Can you push your palms together and hold
for 30 seconds?

Note: Push your palms against each other just hard enough so that
you feel you are doing what is asked. This is not a strength test.

This movement experiment poses the questions: Can you organize yourself to comfortably bear a small amount of pressure
through your shoulders, arms, wrists, hands? Can your arms adapt?
If there is any pain as you create the small pressure of pressing your
hands against each other, stop immediately and decrease the pressure to where you feel no pain/or discomfort. A key idea for adapting successfully to the demands of life is: *If you can find where the
effort is pain-free, you are more likely to feel safe doing physical
activities.* The goal is to help you develop the confidence you need
to eliminate or modify any pain based on how you choose to move.
(This is adaptability.) To put it another way—*you can* explore to find
the amount of effort to get the job done in a reasonable and pain-

free way. Use a mirror to see if you are following the directions and hold this posture for 30 seconds to a minute.

Relevance of movement to daily living: This movement experiment relates to your ability to push to open a door, to support your body weight, to hold up an object in front of you, to carry a tray, to push away as when defending yourself, or to push a grocery cart. These are all common arm, shoulder, and hand activities and are key to a sense of ease, control, and power in organizing your daily life. If you find this movement causes discomfort or pain, begin to explore ways to relax your arms, shoulders, and hands. For example, at rest when you put weight on your hand, be sure the palm is flat (see Figure 20). Many times if you rest with the hand using fingertip pressure, more tension will occur at the shoulder and neck (see Figure 21). (Refer to "Sitting," p. 18, for more cues). Remember to explore the movements and positions that are suggested. The goal is to adjust to find the easiest way, and if you cannot find comfort, ask your physician or physical therapist for advice.

3. Twisting and Reaching Using Your Arms, Shoulders, Chest, and Spine

FUNCTIONAL QUESTION: Can you *reach one hand over the same shoulder* and the other hand behind your back and allow your fingertips to touch? Is this easier with the right hand reaching over the right shoulder, or if you switch and do it with the left hand reaching over the left shoulder? (See Figures 22 and 23.) (Use the "Rate Yourself" score sheet.)

Rate yourself: 1. feels natural; 2. can do but with effort; 3. can do but irritates; 4. can do but causes pain; 5. cannot do/choose not to do.

Common signs of trying too hard, overuse, or fatigue: Strain felt in the shoulder area, elevating the shoulders, rounding the upper back, tightening the entire chest, alterations in the ease of sitting, or holding your breath.

Hints to improve Natural Ease™: Sit with Natural Ease™ and use props (pillows or towels) as needed. Place one hand on the side of your neck and slide it along to feel your entire shoulder and back up to the base of your neck. If there is no discomfort, slide the hand down your back and gently stroke from side to side to find how far you can easily slide the fingertips down your back. If you can do this in a slow and comfortable manner, let that arm rest in that position (hand on same shoulder, fingertips pointing down) while sliding your other hand along your waistband or belt and gently stroking your back with the back of your hand (the side opposite the palm of your hand). If it still feels comfortable, slowly slide the back of this hand up the back of the chest and allow the fingertips of both hands to meet. Breathe normally.

This movement experiment measures the ability of your upper body to adapt. If it is not possible for your fingers to touch, it means that vigorous contact athletics may not be safe at this time. The lack of ability for the upper chest and arms to move into unusual patterns places the requirement to move quickly to the right or left on other parts of the body such as the legs, the hips, and the lower back and increases the risk of strain, injury, or overuse. Movement works in a chain of effort, and if your chest (rib cage musculature) is tight and does not move easily, it means that other parts of your body will need to do extra work that they were not designed for. It is desirable for the upper body and arms to participate naturally in vigorous motions such as running/jumping. Even in casual walking, the motion of swinging the arms is natural, helpful, and necessary to allow walking to occur with the natural participation of the neck, shoulders, and chest and the lower back, hips, and knees. In a sense, the movement of the arms, the shoulders, and the upper chest is leading the lower back, the hips, and the knees in a movement that is safe and easy on each part of the body that is involved. Try to put this to use in daily life. The upper body is a cooperating partner in movement with the lower body and the legs for walking, running, and jumping.

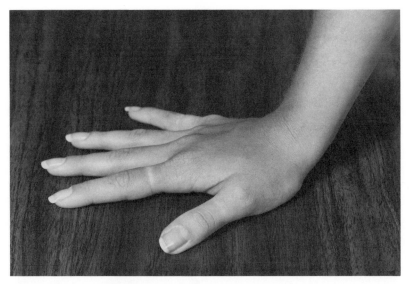

Figure 20. Palm flat to support weight.

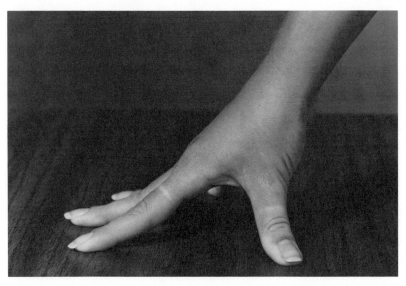

Figure 21. Using spider position to support weight can increase arm, shoulder, and neck tension.

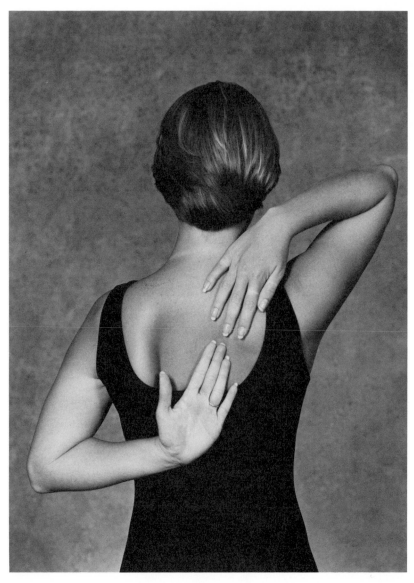

Figure 22. Can you reach your right hand over your right shoulder and
touch your left hand as it reaches from
behind your back?

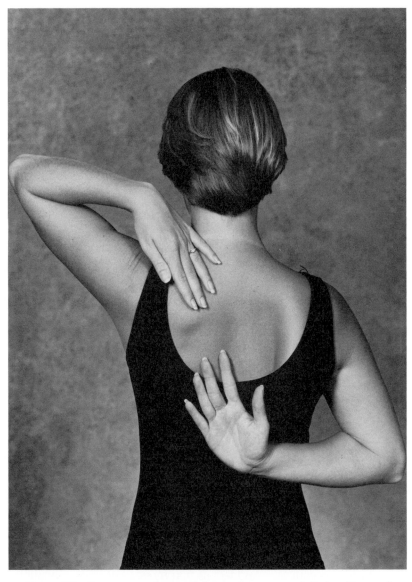

Figure 23. Can you reach your left hand over your left shoulder and touch your right hand as it reaches from behind your back?

Relevance of movement to daily living: The upper body motions are key in desk work. If the upper body (chest) is rigid, it is likely that either the arms and/or the neck will need to overwork to compensate. It is important that the upper body be able to adapt naturally. The natural chain of movement involves easy, natural motion of the arms, the shoulders, the neck, the chest, and the lower body. In daily life, this can mean reaching under the car seat or behind the couch to pick up an object. Mechanical repairs on all types of large engines can often require a twisting and reaching motion of the arms, shoulders, chest, and spine.

4. Relaxing the Face, Neck, and Jaw

FUNCTIONAL QUESTION: Can you *slowly, gently slide your lower jaw forward* and park your lower teeth in front of your upper teeth? Can you relax your facial muscles in this position? Can you breathe naturally in this position? (See Figure 24.) (Use the "Rate Yourself" score sheet.)

Rate yourself: 1. feels natural; 2. can do but with effort; 3. can do but irritates; 4. can do but causes pain; 5. cannot do/choose not to do.

Common signs of trying too hard, overuse, or fatigue: Tightening your neck and moving your head forward, tightening your chest, holding your breath, or clenching your jaw.

Hints to improve Natural Ease™: Sit as described earlier with your jaw relaxed and your teeth not touching. Move your tongue gently in and out a half inch (very small motion). Do the tongue motion slowly; rest by breathing in and breathing out once between each time you move your tongue barely out of your mouth and back in again. If there is no pain or discomfort while doing this, place your hands on your face and feel as you move your lower jaw a little to the right, rest in that position and take in a breath and let it out, then move your lower jaw a little to the left, rest in that position and take in a breath and let it out, and then rest. If there is no pain, gen-

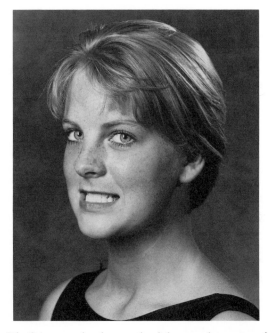

Figure 24. Can you slowly, gently slide your lower jaw forward and park your lower teeth in front of your upper teeth?

tly slide your lower jaw a little forward and place your bottom teeth in front of your upper teeth (see Figure 24).[1]

Do not continue the movement if it is painful. If you discover major restrictions, tightness, discomfort, or actual pain, contact your local physical therapist, physician, or dentist, as this will be an early warning sign of possible difficulties. It is recommended that you seek out a clinician who specializes in temporomandibular joint (TMJ) and head and neck movement problems if chewing is painful. It is assumed that chewing is okay for you.

Relevance of movement to daily living: The ability to open your mouth for talking, shouting, or other types of communication is a basic social skill. The ability to open your mouth to brush your teeth and to perform other dental care is also critical. The ability to open your mouth to allow the dentist to repair a cavity is also a necessary function. Natural jaw motions are needed to chew and eat without pain and therefore essential to your life functions.[1]

5. Sitting and Bending: Reaching Using Your Spine, Arms, Pelvis, and Legs

FUNCTIONAL QUESTION: Total body flexibility (use the "Rate Yourself" score sheet).

- Step 1: In sitting, can you take one leg and cross it and lay the ankle comfortably on the other thigh (see Figure 25)? If that is easy and pain free, proceed to step 2. If not, stop the movement experiment and just read the rest of this segment.

- Step 2: Place one thumb on your chin and point your index finger down toward the foot with the ankle resting on your other thigh. Lean forward and, using the other hand to help, try to move the leg on your lap so that your index finger touches the lowest part of your heel, the side of your foot, or your big toe (see Figure 26). Proceed to the next step only if the previous movements are pain free.

- Step 3: Can you touch your chin to your heel or big toe (see Figure 27)? Repeat steps 1–3 for your other leg.

Rate yourself: 1. feels natural; 2. can do but with effort; 3. can do but irritates; 4. can do but causes pain; 5. cannot do/choose not to do.

Common signs of trying too hard, overuse, or fatigue: Sitting with your body rolled back and not sitting on your sitting bones. Holding your breath during the movement (your breathing should not be disturbed as you perform any of the movement experiments). You notice tension in your arms, neck, chest, and/or jaw, or clenching your jaw. Note: The entire body does not need to tighten.

Hints to improve Natural Ease™: The task is divided into three parts so you can get to know yourself in a gentle and comfort-

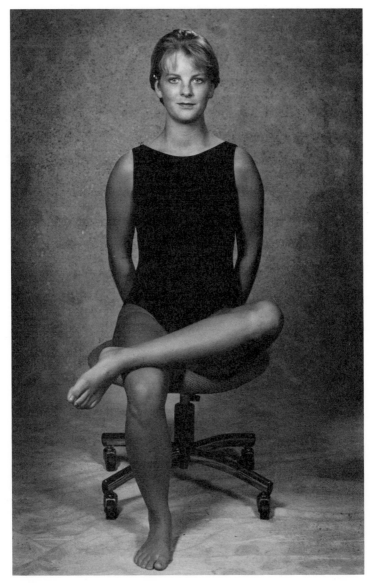

Figure 25. Can you take one leg and cross it—lift it comfortably onto the other thigh?

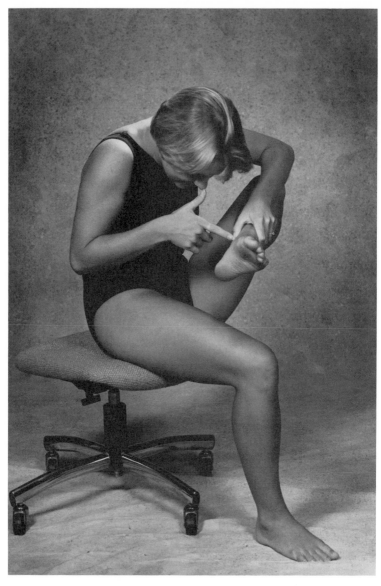

Figure 26. On the same hand, can you touch your nose with the thumb and your foot with the index finger?

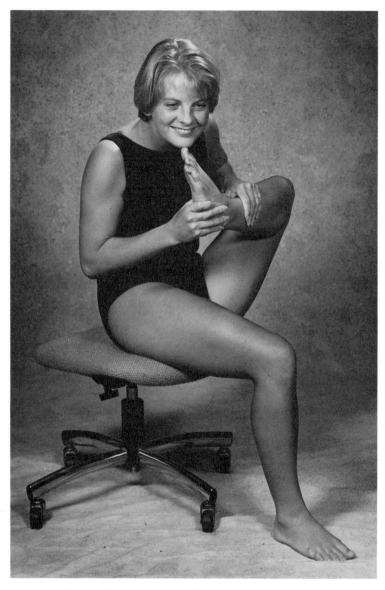

Figure 27. Can you touch your chin to your heel
or big toe?

able manner. Remember, accomplishment is not the key goal. As you get to know what is usual for you, it is then possible to choose to change and work to improve one function, ability, or idea at a time. This experiment is about discovering what is easy for you so that you can start learning to improve by working from a realistic perception of your current abilities. It is important to be aware of what is reasonable so that you can plan a lifelong program of enjoyment and physical/emotional fitness (or, put another way, so that you can avoid constant severe strain in your life). The goal is to make learning new and more efficient movements easy and enjoyable during your entire lifetime.

Human beings can change or modify more easily if *one* aspect or idea is tackled at a time. Before you even think about performing step 1, notice your breathing and where you feel you are breathing. But that doesn't necessarily mean to change your breathing. Just notice what you are doing—"How am I breathing?" As you become aware of what you are doing, you can work toward what you want. *The Natural Ease™ of breathing should not be disturbed as you assess how you move.* You need to continue to breathe in your regular way as you move. If breathing is disturbed during movement, then the movement becomes an emergency function, but this is only necessary for a few seconds in most of our lives. Daily life should involve an ease of motion, with breathing simply happening to support the ongoing well-being of the individual. Breathing needs to occur simultaneously with movement.

The next step is the hip hinge motion (refer to section 1c to review the motion, if necessary). It is presumed that the hip hinge motion is pain free and feels reasonable. If it feels awkward, please proceed with extra caution to step 1. Feel free to use your hands to assist you as you attempt to lift your leg and place the ankle on the opposite thigh. If this motion is not easy, and leaving the leg resting there for 1 minute is not comfortable or reasonable, *STOP—PUT THE LEG DOWN AND DO NOT PROCEED TO THE NEXT*

STEP. The goal is to identify what is reasonably easy. If the first experiment was not easy, it is recommended that you contact your physician or physical therapist, since this limitation in flexibility may lead to walking problems or may decrease your urge to be physically active.

Only proceed to step 2 when step 1 is easy. As you try step 2, be sure that you do it slowly enough that your breathing is not disturbed or altered. If you cannot touch your index finger to your heel, hold a ruler in your fingers and slide it out until you can touch your heel and then easily stay in that position (breathing comfortably) for 30 seconds. Record how many inches of ruler you needed to slide out to touch your heel today. This measurement is a record of your flexibility today. You are adaptable, and with practice you can see the progress or changes that may be possible. Remember, the goal is to learn what is easy for you. Why? *Learning motions that are easy enhances the urge to explore new ways to move.* It is nearly impossible to learn new skills if you are struggling with physical discomfort or holding your breath. If you do strain yourself in this manner, it will be hard to remember later what you've learned, so all of the effort will only serve you for that moment.

Proceed to step 3 only if step 2 is reasonably easy—is worth doing again, feels interesting, and there is no discomfort. A part of you may have an incredible urge to prove to yourself that you are totally perfect in your flexibility. Perfection is an unrealistic state of mind, and if you force yourself, pain is common. Stop using this forceful approach and allow yourself to be what and who you really are. If you truly want improved flexibility/adaptability, go to the end of the book and begin to play with the movement experiments that are presented for the feet and the lower body and refer to the bibliography for references to other books and tapes that can help you learn to move easier. Regardless of whether you are twenty years of age, fifty years of age, or eighty-five years of age, learning is possible and your ability to learn is not limited by how old you are.

After you have done step 2 and it felt okay, you can try the third step. For this experiment, place the same leg on your lap as you used for step 2. This needs to be done in such a way that your breathing *is not disturbed or held.* Touch your big toe to your chin and, holding it in that position, just breathe for 5 seconds and then stop and rest (see Figure 27).

Another way to do step 3 is to lie on the floor on your back or side and perform the same activity. Doing the movement experiment on the floor is simply another version of the third experiment and can be classified as experiment 2.5. The support of the floor can be a help for some people, perhaps because it makes the movement more coordinated and therefore it feels easier. Accept your level of ability today, begin to experiment to refine your movement and your coordination, and gradually become more efficient in your total body flexibility. Repeat steps 1, 2, and 3 for the other leg as appropriate and record your score.

Relevance of movement to daily living: Basic activities of daily living such as cutting your toenails and washing between your toes are directly related to your ability to do the first movement experiment of placing your foot on the thigh of your other leg. What if you have a sliver in your foot and you need to remove it? This activity is similar to the motions that were done for step 2. The third movement experiment represents the ability to curl up and roll, which may be needed when you are pushed off balance and begin to fall. The flexibility to curl and roll with a fall creates a way of protecting the head and the internal organs and minimizes the local injury of one or more of the joints or organs. The movements involve your ability to organize to safely roll when a fall cannot be avoided. Step 3 movements are also needed in almost all contact sports to avoid local joint strain or injury (i.e., knees, groin, collar bones, wrist). The ability to go in the direction of the unexpected force in a coordinated way can give you some element of control, and therefore there is increased safety. (Think of the athletes who dive to reach the ball and roll into the end zone—if they did not roll, the impact would be severe and could potentially cause a strain or injury.) The movements in the third experiment are useful in contact sports and if a fall or accident cannot be avoided as a part of real life.

6. Supporting the Body Weight Using Arms, Legs, Neck, and Spine

FUNCTIONAL QUESTION:

6a. Can you get down on the floor from a chair to a hands-and-knees position?

6b. Can you stand on your hands and knees for 1 minute? Note: Your hands are below your shoulders, your knees are below your hips. (See Figure 28.)

Use the "Rate Yourself" score sheet.

Rate yourself: 1. feels natural; 2. can do but with effort; 3. can do but irritates; 4. can do but causes pain; 5. cannot do/choose not to do.

Common signs of trying too hard, overuse, or fatigue: Holding your breath, tightening your chest, neck, or legs and feet. If your knees feel tender, feel free to use pillows under each knee. If your wrists are tender, lean on your entire forearm as well as your hands, instead of just your hands and wrists. If modifications do not produce a pain-free position, stop the activity immediately and contact your local physical therapist or physician for further problem solving.

Hints to improve Natural Ease™: It is acceptable to use hockey knee pads or gardening knee pads to make your knees feel comfortable. Getting down on all fours can present a challenge. If you feel the need for support, use a stable object to lean on (i.e., a countertop or a chair braced firmly against a wall). Lean on the chair or other object and slowly bend one knee and lower yourself to the floor. It is acceptable to lean on the back or the seat of the chair, whichever is most comfortable for you.

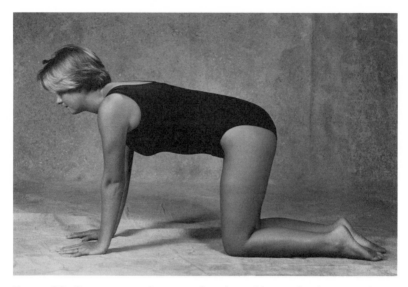

Figure 28. Can you stand on your hands and knees for 1 minute (comfortably)?

Now slowly push the chair away and place one hand on the floor at a time. Breathe normally. Allow your head to hang down comfortably.

6c. Can you curl your entire back up toward the ceiling? The goal is to try to involve your entire spine in the Natural Ease™ of efficient movement. Can you find a comfortable mid-position of rest for your back as you stand on your hands and knees?

Use the "Rate Yourself" score sheet.

Check that your feet and lower legs are relaxed and feel supple to you. No tightness or effort is needed in the lower part of the leg in this position. Check one leg at a time; it is easier to pay attention to only one part of the body at a time.

Relevance of movement to daily living: The ability to use the position on all fours is a critical safety factor in case of a fire. Smoke rises, so it is important that you be able to crawl to safety, breathing the least-polluted air. The ability to get down on all fours is also useful for picking up objects that fall on the floor. The most common activity is simply helping yourself get up from the floor if you happen to fall down. But, you protest, "I never fall down." Well, most adults do fall once every few years. Some people fall as often as once or twice a year. If I know I can safely get up if I do fall in the snow, on the ice, or on a wet surface, I will be less afraid of falling. The more afraid I am of falling, the tighter my body will be as I walk, and this increases the chances for falling. The ability to get up from the floor gives you increased confidence about your safety, especially if you live alone. Many ball sports involve the activity of getting down to the ground (to pick up the ball). Pleasant activities on hands and knees involve things like playing with small children or gardening. Practical activities include washing or waxing floors and many types of home repair.

7. Looking with Eyes, Neck, Chest, and Spine

FUNCTIONAL QUESTION: While standing on all fours, can you look up and down with comfort and ease? Can you look to the right and the left? Your palms should be flat and the pressure equal on your hands and knees (natural hip width apart). (See Figures 29, 30, and 31.) (Use the "Rate Yourself" score sheet.)

Rate yourself: 1. feels natural; 2. can do but with effort; 3. can do but irritates; 4. can do but causes pain; 5. cannot do/choose not to do.

Common signs of trying too hard, overuse, or fatigue: Holding your breath, clenching your teeth and jaw, moving your eyes and head as one unit instead of letting your eyes lead the movement of your head. Moving your head, neck, and chest as a unit instead of letting your eyes lead, your head follow, and then perhaps, if you turn even farther, your neck and your chest can also participate in the movement.

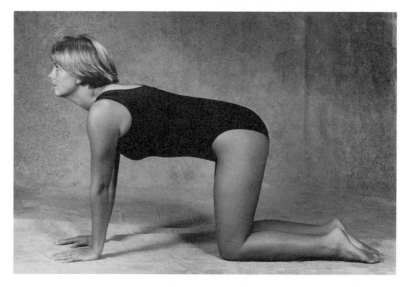

Figure 29. Can you look up?

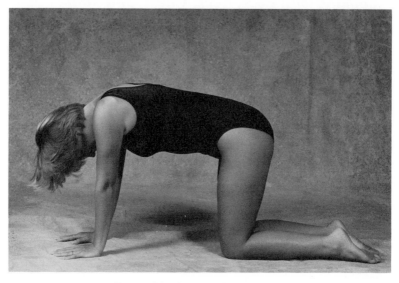

Figure 30. Can you look down?

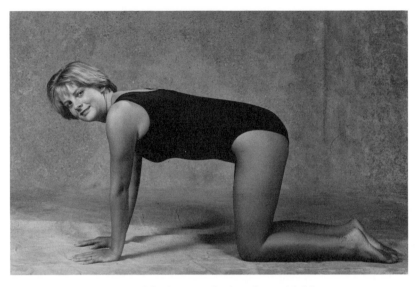

Figure 31. Can you look right and left?

Hints to improve Natural Ease™: While on all fours, you need to be comfortable in the starting position, and if being on all fours is not comfortable for you, try leaning on your forearms to do the head-turning experiment. Note: If you cannot get comfortable on all fours, skip this movement and circle a "5" on the score sheet.

Check that breathing is natural. Allow your stomach to be supported by gravity, which is the opposite of sucking it in. Do not suck in your stomach in this position; just let it hang suspended. Allow your eyes by themselves to glance gently to the right and then to the left. If moving your eyes alone creates a feeling of pressure in your eyes or head, stop the activity. Try to do a smaller, gentler motion to glance with just your eyes. If you can find an easy way, then proceed. If you notice that moving your eyes is not easy, then stop the experiment. If there is pressure in your eyes or head as you glance right and left, it means you are using $20 worth of effort to glance when a $10 motion would get the job done safely. Do less.

Coordination of movement means using only the minimum of effort. It is usually by doing a little less that you can begin to improve ease of motion. The eyes are totally equipped to move with ease, and there is no need to make movement an incredible effort. Breathing is not to be disturbed by eye movement. If you hold your breath to move your eyes, you are saying, "This is an emergency activity." It is not meant to be that way. Allow your eyes to glance gently to the right and then let your head also begin to turn to the right (if you want to look further), and lastly, allow your shoulder to move slightly back and around in that direction. Repeat the same activity to your left. Allow your eyes to lead and let your head and neck very consciously follow the motion of your eyes; let the movement be very gentle. Try to decrease your effort to only 50 percent of the effort that you just expended. What if you went at half the speed so that you moved more slowly than on the first attempt? See what happens if you simply slow down the speed of the movement by 50 percent. What if you make the movement 50 percent smaller? This means that if you turned your head to be able to see something almost to the side of you, just turn your head so that you get only halfway to that same place the next time. Discover what is easy. Take pleasure in movements that are easy. Get to know yourself and what feels easy for you.

Relevance of movement to daily living: The ease of movement of the eyes to quickly assess a situation by looking is essential to survival. If a person intends to attack you or steal your money, they would prefer to attack an individual who looks straight ahead or someone who appears unable to move their head easily to follow the movement of their eyes to the right and left. In your outdoor activities, a rapid look to avoid a flying object is also critical for safety. The eyes, head, and neck need to move as an easy chain of events. The arms need to be free to catch you as you fall to protect your face. Your eyes and arms working together are important to adapting, feeling confident, and being safe in real-life situations.

8. Organizing the Spine, Pelvis, Knees, Ankles, and Feet To Sit and Rest

CAUTION: This movement experiment presumes that a starting position on all fours is comfortable. Do not try this experiment if you have discomfort standing on all fours.

FUNCTIONAL QUESTION:

8a. From all fours, can you move back and sit on a firm cushion that is 12 inches high placed on top of your heels and on top of your lower leg and rest pain free for 30 to 60 seconds? (See Figure 32.)

8b. If you lower the cushion to 8 inches, can you sit for 30 to 60 seconds comfortably? (See Figure 33.) Proceed to the next experiment only if you feel no pulling, pressure, or pain. *Do not* cause a feeling of pulling, pressure, or pain.

8c. Presuming that parts 8a and 8b felt easy to perform, lower the cushion to 6 inches, to 4 inches, and to 2 inches for 30 to 60 seconds each, and then use no pillow at all for 60 seconds. (See Figure 34.)

Rate yourself: 1. feels natural; 2. can do but with effort; 3. can do but irritates; 4. can do but causes pain; 5. cannot do/choose not to do.

Common signs of trying too hard, overuse, or fatigue: Avoid holding your breath, tightening your toes and feet to control the motion, and rounding of your lower or upper back. Note: The focus of movement needs to be in the hips, the trunk, the pelvis, and the knees.

Hints to improve Natural Ease™: As you kneel, it is presumed that this position is comfortable. If you know or think that you have sensitive knees, then place a soft pad under your knees. It is presumed that your upper body is relaxed with the head and shoulders at ease and the weight resting on the lower body. A

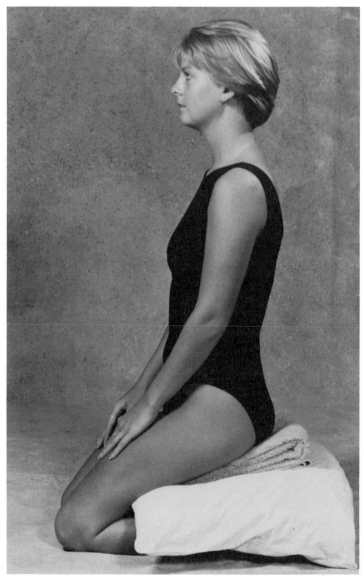

Figure 32. Can you sit on 12 inches of firm support resting on top of your heels (30–60 seconds)?

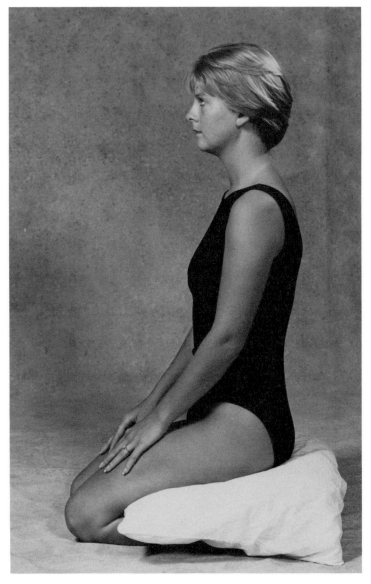

Figure 33. Can you sit on 8 inches of firm support for
30–60 seconds?

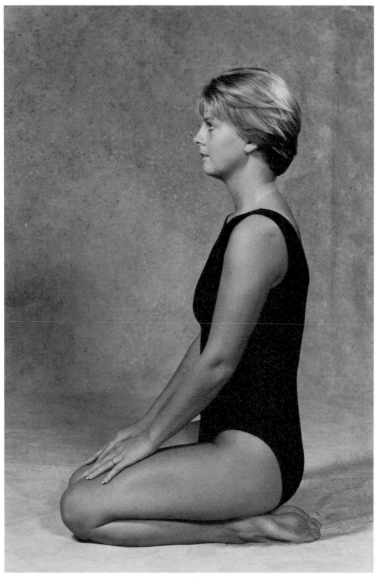

Figure 34. Can you sit on your heels?

strange idea? It is important that your head and body are neither in front and nor in back of your hips (just held naturally above them). If needed, place your hands on a sofa or a coffee table to control the ease of lowering to sit on the cushion for each experiment. Breathing needs to be natural and undisturbed.

You may notice that the top of your foot and shin are pulling, hurting, or otherwise irritated and interfering with the ease of sitting on your heels. In this case, you will need to use a cushion or pillow to increase your comfort. Place the pillow or cushion under your ankles in a place that supports them and relieves the pain and pulling (see Figure 35). A small 6-inch by 6-inch or 8-inch by 8-inch feather pillow works well to mold to the tender areas and let you learn to relax. It may help to experiment where to place the pillow and how much padding you really need to get to your "easy learning" position. Only proceed to the next movement experiment when it feels easy to sit on a 12-inch cushion without a small pillow under your ankles. One goal is to discover how to relax the muscles so you need less support under the ankles, or none at all.

As you do the movement experiment, let one hand feel what your feet and toes are doing as you lower yourself from kneeling to sit on the 12-inch cushion. Your toes need to relax and not tighten as you lower yourself to sit. Now it is time to talk to yourself. As your hand is on your feet, be thinking: "My feet and ankles do not need to tighten in order to lower myself to sit on the cushion. On the contrary, this is the exact opposite of what is useful and supportive for me to really do the activity in a coordinated fashion." You might discover that your toes have "run away" from you—that they tighten every time you attempt to sit back on the 12-inch cushion. If that is the case, you should contact your physician or physical therapist and share the results of this assessment. A simple yoga class, relaxation training, or Feldenkrais class, or working with a physical therapist, may minimize your chances of foot, ankle, knee, or hip problems and increase your enjoyment for walking. Remember, causing yourself pain to prove you can move is a useless effort.

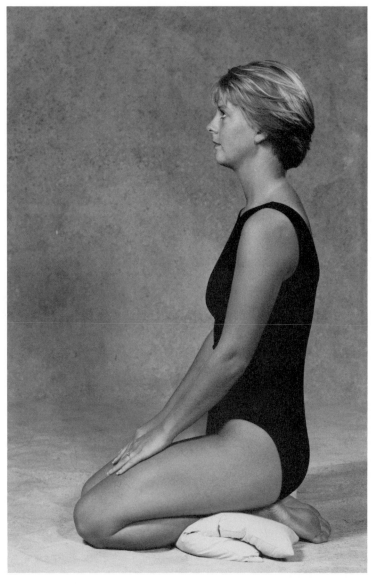

Figure 35. If your ankles are uncomfortable, try placing a soft support under them (temporarily).

You are a valuable, worthwhile person who is playing with these ideas to learn to adapt better to the movements needed for daily activities (to carry out the tasks that are important to you).

Relevance of movement to daily living: If you can sit comfortably on your heels, then gardening and all work that you do in this position (brick laying, cement work, etc.) can be less strenuous. It is presumed that your head would be above your hips if you are sitting upright.

It is also important to consider that the ability to both get down on the floor to pick up something or to get yourself up off the floor is greatly influenced by ease of movement in your lower back, hips, thighs, knees, ankles, and feet. As your confidence in your movement abilities increases, you will enjoy walking, sitting, and standing activities and feel safer in action. The goal is to carry out desired activities with Natural Ease™.

If you find restrictions, it means that you are not going to be efficient in moving and you will increase your chances of getting hurt or having an accident. If your body is tight at rest, you will not enjoy doing activities as much, and the urge to move will lessen. Note: As you go through the motions in this section, when you feel tired or any minor strain, stop. A good resting position is with the forehead on a pillow (see Figure 36). If this position is not restful, then roll to the side and lie down on the floor to rest.

9. Reaching When Sitting

FUNCTIONAL QUESTION: Can you sit on the floor or bed with your knees straight and legs out in front of you without any discomfort or pulling (for 1 minute)? If you can answer yes to step 1, proceed to the next step.

9a. Can you lean forward with both your arms as if to touch your toes without bending your knees? If it is reasonably

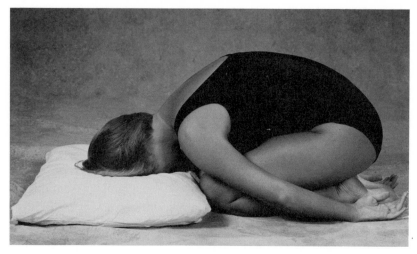

Figure 36. Rest your forehead on a pillow or on the floor.

easy, and your hands can actually touch your toes and *your knees are still straight,* proceed to the next step. (See Figure 37.)

9b. Can you reach beyond your toes? (See Figure 38.)

Use the "Rate Yourself" score sheet.

Rate yourself: 1. 1+ inch beyond toes; 2. touch toes; 3. 1+ inch less than touch toes; 4. 2+ inches less than touch toes; 5. 3+ inches less than touch toes.

Common signs of trying too hard, overuse, or fatigue: The first experiment is to sit and then straighten your knees. If you cannot do this or you catch yourself holding your breath, then move more slowly. "But," you say, "I like to go fast—that's who I am." Since you know how to do a fast movement, then why not learn *how to enjoy moving more slowly.* If you want different results, you may have to do things in a different way. There are times in life when going slowly is the only safe way to relate to other people and to yourself.

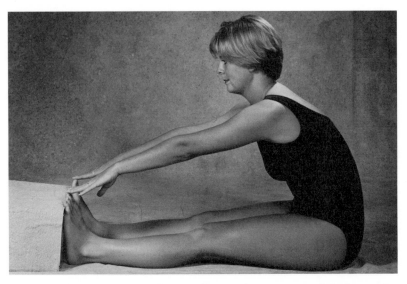

Figure 37. Sitting on the floor or firm surface, can you lean forward (knees not bending) to touch your toes? (Bending occurs primarily at hips and pelvic area.)

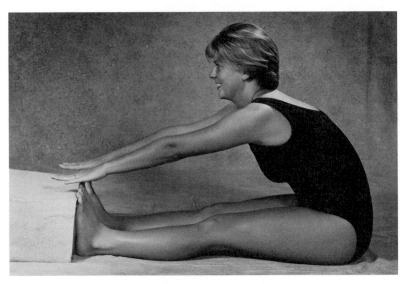

Figure 38. Can you reach beyond your toes?

Bending your knees is the most common error. If you need to bend your knees in order to feel comfortable, then the experiment cannot give you valid information to learn more about yourself. If you cannot go beyond step 1, then read the hints to increase ease and explore how to increase your coordination, and repeat this movement experiment later.

Hints to improve Natural Ease™: You may have looked at the figures and are saying to yourself, "This is not me." *Don't* give in and not try. A way to help yourself is to try to sit on a 2- to 3-inch cushion. Does using a cushion allow you to sit and straighten your knees? Check that your legs are hip width apart—holding your feet close together can cause an unnaturally strenuous movement. If sitting this way feels okay, take your hands and slide them down your legs as far as you can do so easily. If you can breathe and touch your toes, stop and rest. Breathe in that position with your hands touching your toes. Sit up and then try to reach for your toes again by sliding your hands down your legs as you continue to breathe naturally. Do not interrupt your breathing to explore your ability to move. Experiment with resting in a position 10 percent less than your best so you can truly relax and enjoy the position.

Relevance of movement to daily living: The movements involved to make this action easy are also involved in walking or in riding a horse. Although you may not be a horseback rider, it is important to remember that your lower back is supported by your feet every time you take a step. The free and easy interaction between the feet and the lower back is crucial to be able to walk and enjoy walking and, more importantly, running. "But I'm not a runner," you say. The most convincing argument I can make to encourage you to learn to live with ease is that your lower back and pelvis are directly connected to the pleasure and ease of sexual expression. You will never know what you are missing until you discover how to let your entire body participate in the movements of sexual activity. (Note: Movement is only a small part of sexual pleasure; other factors can include the love, caring, commitment, and mutual respect between the two partners, etc.)

FUNCTIONAL QUESTION:

9c. Can you get up from the floor without help?

Use the "Rate Yourself" score sheet.

Hints to improve Natural Ease™: It is time to get up off the floor. When you are ready, move to a half-kneeling position (one knee and the other foot on the ground or floor, as in Figure 39), rest, and then get a firm grip on a stable object for support. Leverage can help you to get up more easily. Instead of pushing straight up (which is very hard on the knees), try to use the strategy pictured in Figure 40. Pivot backward to straighten the knee of the foot that is flat on the floor. From this position, simply step forward with the leg in back and gently straighten yourself (see Figure 41).

10. Balance

PRELIMINARY QUESTION: Can you stand on the floor with your feet flat and lean forward until you feel your toes grip slightly (motion occurs mostly at ankles and toes)? Only if this is easy should you proceed to the activity on the trampoline. (See Figures 42a and 42b.)

FUNCTIONAL QUESTION:

10a. Can you stand on two feet on a trampoline and feel safe? Only proceed if the answer is yes; otherwise stop. Can you stand and lean on the trampoline the same way as you did on the floor? (See Figures 43 and 44.)

10b. Hold onto a stable object as you try to shift ~~the majority~~ *most* of your weight forward, but leave *both feet flat* on the mat of the trampoline the entire time.

Use the "Rate Yourself" score sheet.

Rate yourself: 1. feels natural; 2. can do but with effort; 3. can do but irritates; 4. can do but causes pain; 5. cannot do/choose not to do.

10c. Can you stand with ~~the majority~~ *most* of your weight on your right foot (both feet still flat on the mat)? (If necessary, hold onto an object for support.)

10d. Can you stand with ~~the majority~~ *most* of your weight on your left foot?

10e. Can you bounce yourself with both feet flat on the trampoline?

NOTE: Only do the weight shift if it feels safe to proceed. Can you stand quietly on a trampoline with your feet flat using two hands for support? Can you stand with your feet flat and rock yourself up and down (head moving closer to the ceiling and away from the ceiling)? Try using only one hand to support yourself on a counter or railing. If this feels natural and easy, then try it without using either hand for support! If this feels natural and easy, only then try to bounce with no hand support and rate how this feels. (See Figure 44.)

NOTE: Only proceed to the last movement experiment if bouncing without using your hands for support felt easy.

10f. Can you bounce yourself and let both heels lift slightly off the mat of the trampoline? (Use the "Rate Yourself" score sheet.) Can you bounce up and down and let both heels lift slightly off the mat of the trampoline using two-handed support? If this feels easy and natural, then try it with one-handed support. If this feels easy, try it without using either hand for support.

10g. Can you bounce on the trampoline and alternate heel contact (begin with two-handed support and if that is reasonably easy, try it with one-handed support, and finally, if that is reasonably easy, without using either hand for support and with an upright posture)? (See Figure 45.)

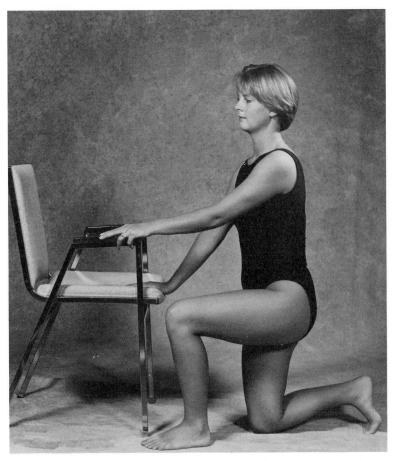

Figure 39. Can you get back up from the floor without help?

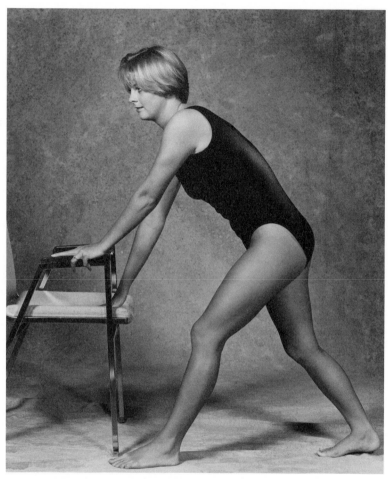

Figure 40. Pivot backward to straighten the leg with the foot flat on the floor and in front.

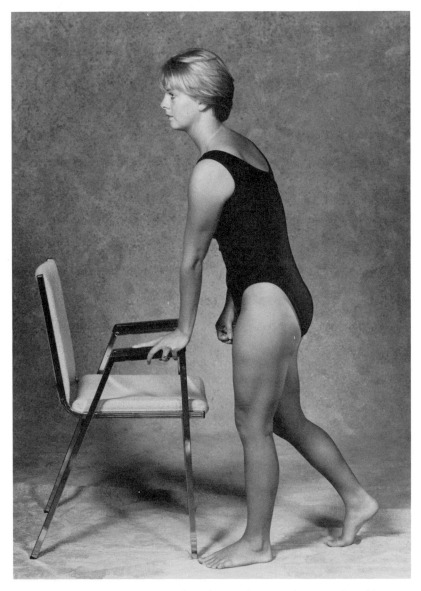

Figure 41. Move the back foot forward to stand up comfortably.

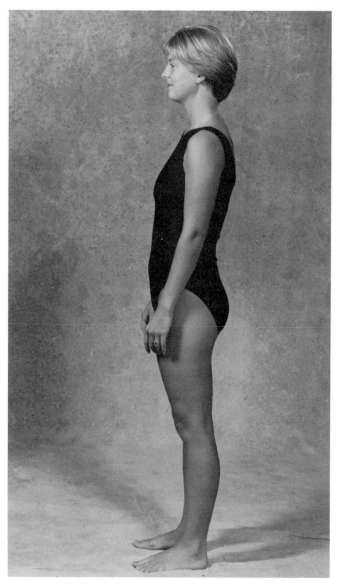

Figure 42a. Stand relaxed on the floor.

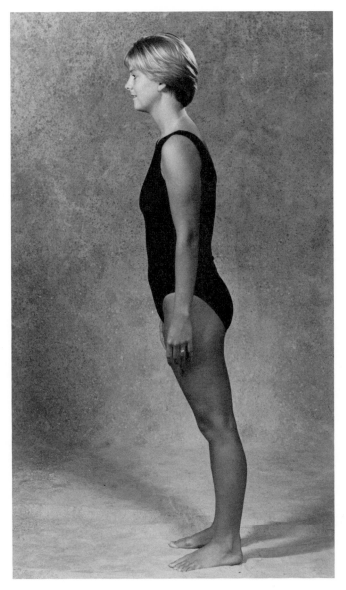

Figure 42b. Lean forward from your ankles until you feel your toes grip slightly into the floor.

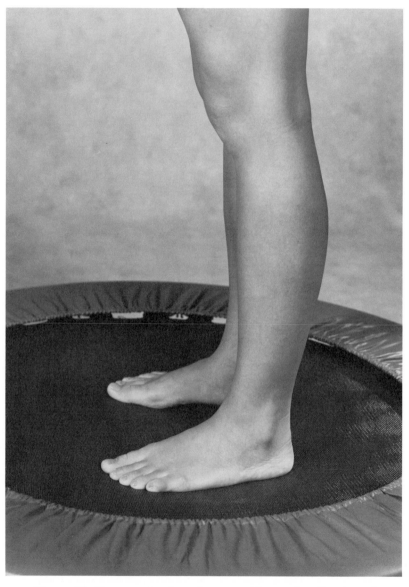

Figure 43. Can you stand on the mat with your feet flat (equal pressure on heels and front of foot)?

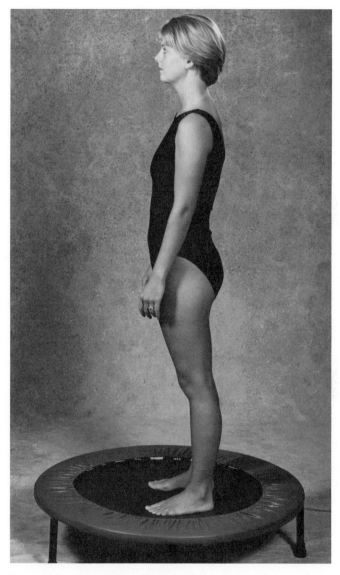

Figure 44. Can you lean forward from your ankles until you feel your toes grip slightly into the mat of the trampoline? If that feels natural, try bouncing up and down but keeping your feet flat on the mat.

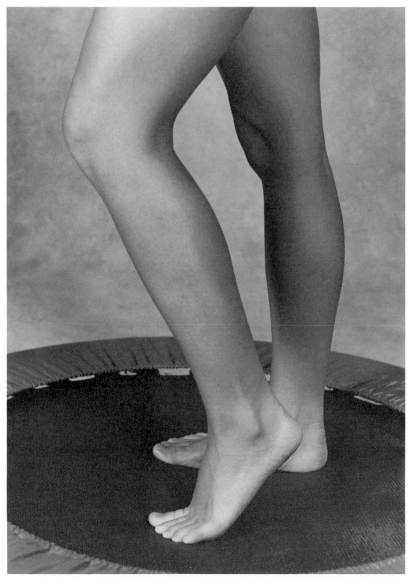

Figure 45. Can you alternately shift the weight from your right foot to your left foot?

Common signs of trying too hard, overuse, or fatigue: Holding the breath is the most common error noted. As you move to shift your weight, your entire body needs to be participating gently with no local areas of tightness. Holding the rib cage stiff is another common problem, as is looking down or locking the arms and creating a fist with the hands.

Hints to increase Natural Ease™: Do less than you feel you can. In other words, don't give 100 percent effort. Balance is like stacking blocks on each other. If you go slowly and move gently, you can stack more blocks on top of each other. If you feel you need to hold on to stand and bounce on the trampoline, then I would say it is not a place for you to learn to balance with ease. You will have to work too hard, and the risk will be too much of a distraction to you. Get off the trampoline and put a small cushion on the floor and stand on it. Find an activity from the list above that does not require you to support yourself with your hands to feel safe. "But," you say, "I cannot really do any of these movements and feel safe unless I hold on." Guess what? This is good news. Why? Because now you know how to create the setting for learning. As you learn to improve your balance, it will feel good and you will want to learn more. Concern for safety is a healthy human response, and it controls the fear of falling and decreases the risk of falling.

How can you learn to balance better? You need to start where it is reasonably easy. Sit down on a chair. Let me introduce you to your feet. Why? If you begin to experiment with your feet, your pelvis, and your lower back, it will give you new ideas for moving well and assist you in developing better balance (see Chapter IV for sample foot experiments and the hints to improve ease of sitting at the beginning of this chapter). The goal—learning to balance so the skeleton does the primary work of supporting your weight and the muscles are free to do the moving of the body.

Relevance of movements to daily living: Balance is used for all activities of daily living, including sitting, kneeling, standing, reaching, walking, running, jumping, etc. At work or at play, adequate balance is needed to feel safe and effective in action. The ability to balance is built on a willingness to risk trying to find out what you can do with Natural Ease™. As you use these ideas, the hope is that you will know how to create a way to promote lifelong learning.

Life will keep providing unpredictable changes (big and small). The goal is to create a response in yourself that matches the demands of the task to be mastered. As each of us learns how to adapt using our whole self in a free and easy way, new goals and dreams can develop. How? Think about the person who sits and looks ahead and is not in the habit of turning to look to the right or to the left. They will get less information about the world around them than the person who can turn and is in the habit of looking over their shoulder and allowing the majority *most* of their body to participate in movement. The more you spread the effort of moving throughout your body, the less wear and tear there is on each little part of yourself. Help your tired neck by letting your chest and pelvis participate as you turn to look. If you turn to look with greater ease, your dreams and ideas can be better suited to the tasks at hand. You will be better able to balance each demand with a response that is suitable.

Lifelong learning is an idea whose time has come. Change is the ongoing ingredient in real life; therefore, adaptability in the mind (your ideas) and in your body (your flexibility) is needed to have a sense of control over your life. *Enjoy the learning.* If you do not enjoy the learning, it will fall out of your brain tomorrow since it was forced in there and no welcoming arms were there to hold onto the ideas. Experiment with moving and learning so the results are felt by your entire self. As you efficiently adapt to do each task, you will enjoy the new challenges and be ready for more new ones tomorrow.

As a place to begin learning to enhance Natural Ease™, Chapter IV presents a movement lesson for the feet and pelvis. Enjoy your learning!

Reference

1. Reese, M.; Zemach–Bersin, D.; and Mosnontz, C. "TMJ Health-Sensory Motor Exercises for Mouth and Jaw Health," (audio cassette tapes), Sensory Motor Learning Systems, CA, 1988.

Score Sheet

RATE YOURSELF

Can I move to get the job done?
GENERAL MUSCULOSKELETAL SCREENING (Voluntary)

Please circle the appropriate number/word: 1 = feels natural; 2. = can do but with effort; 3 = can do but irritates; 4 = can do but causes pain; 5 = cannot do/choose not to do.

Movement Experiments

1a.	Sitting—is that easy? (3 minutes—no backrest)	1	2	3	4	5
1b.	Sitting in a neutral pelvic tilt (natural arch in back at belt line)	1	2	3	4	5
1c.	Hip hinge—lean forward bending only at hips?	1	2	3	4	5
2.	Push palms together for 30 seconds? (sitting)	1	2	3	4	5
3.	Reach one hand over same shoulder to meet other hand reaching behind back and allow fingertips to touch? (sitting) • Right hand over shoulder • Left hand over shoulder	1 1	2 2	3 3	4 4	5 5
4.	Place lower teeth in front of upper teeth? (sitting)	1	2	3	4	5
5.	Sitting : (a) ankle rests on other thigh; (b) thumb to nose—touch index finger of same hand to inside ankle bone of bent leg; (c) bring one foot to chin with help of arms? a. Left: (a) 1 2 3 4 5 (b) 1 2 3 4 5 (c) 1 2 3 4 5 b. Right: (a) 1 2 3 4 5 (b) 1 2 3 4 5 (c) 1 2 3 4 5					
6a.	Get down on floor?	1	2	3	4	5
6b.	Stand on hands and knees? (30 seconds)	1	2	3	4	5
6c.	Curl up back like a cat?	1	2	3	4	5
7a.	Look up?	1	2	3	4	5
7b.	Let head hang down?	1	2	3	4	5
7c.	Look to your right?	1	2	3	4	5
7d.	Look to your left?	1	2	3	4	5
8a.	Sit back with 12-inch firm cushion on heels—forefoot flat?	1	2	3	4	5
8b.	Sit back with 8-inch firm cushion on heels—forefoot flat?	1	2	3	4	5
8c.	Sit back on heels—forefoot flat?	1	2	3	4	5
9a.	Sit on floor, legs straight, and reach toward toes. Score: 1 = 1+ inch beyond toes; 2 = touch toes; 3 = short of toes by 1 inch; 4 = short by 2 inches; 5 = short by 3 inches	1	2	3	4	5
9b.	Breathe and rest touching toes for 1 minute. (Note: Skip if unable to touch toes—score 5.)	1	2	3	4	5
9c.	Get up from floor without help?	1	2	3	4	5

RATE YOURSELF (continued)

10a.	Stand upright at rest on trampoline. (5–10 seconds)					
	• Need support*	1	2	3	4	5
	• No support*	1	2	3	4	5
10b.	On trampoline, stand and lean forward with feet flat (feel toes slightly grip mat).*	1	2	3	4	5
10c.	On trampoline, stand on two feet but with majority of weight on right foot.*	1	2	3	4	5
10d.	On trampoline, stand on two feet but with majority of weight on left foot.*	1	2	3	4	5
10e.	Can bounce with feet flat on trampoline.					
	• Two-handed support*	1	2	3	4	5
	• One-handed support*.	1	2	3	4	5
	• No support*	1	2	3	4	5
10f.	Can bounce and let both heels lift slightly off mat of trampoline.					
	• Two-handed support*	1	2	3	4	5
	• One-handed support*	1	2	3	4	5
	• No support*	1	2	3	4	5
10g.	Can bounce, alternating heel contact. Note: Only perform if 10e and 10f can be done with no support and upright posture.					
	• Two-handed support*	1	2	3	4	5
	• One-handed support*	1	2	3	4	5
	• No support*	1	2	3	4	5

*If not rated a 1 or 2, stop and score all remaining items a 5.

Scoring:

40–50: Congratulations; your general flexibility is ready to help you at work and at play. For ongoing fitness and well-being, you need to select fitness activities you enjoy doing. It is especially helpful to use cardiovascular/aerobic fitness (i.e., walking, running, dancing, swimming) and coordination/balance/relaxation training/flexibility (i.e., Tai Chi, Yoga, Feldenkrais®, singing, meditation). To help develop your curiosity and fun, try to learn one new movement skill per year.

51–66: Your flexibility may be adequate for activities of daily living. To be active in sports/strenuous work, it is helpful to enhance your flexibility/cardiovascular fitness by such activities as:
- Relaxation training, 5–10 minutes per day;
- Coordination/balance/flexibility training, 5–15 minutes per day;
- Enjoyable cardiovascular activities, 3–4 times per week for 12–20 minutes.

67–85: Stop and reflect. Once you are over 18 years of age, it is time to develop problem-solving skills. It is time to realize that brute strength and speed cannot accomplish every goal. There is a place in life for rest and gentle, timely responses. Contact your doctor, have a thorough physical, and then work with a resource person (i.e., counselor, physical therapist, or support group, as appropriate for you) to discover how to tackle life and use all your talents (mind, body, and spirit). It is important that you learn not to rely too much on the body alone to get the job done. Sample activities for fitness and health promotion include:

1. Identifying a resource person to assist you in enhancing your overall fitness and well-being.

2. Developing an individual health and fitness plan to carry out 12–20 minutes a day as part of daily living (cardiac/coordination/flexibility).

3. For recreation/relaxation, select one or more activities that you enjoy. It is critical to make a commitment to spend 15–30 minutes at physical activities, two to three times a week. Take some time to develop a recreation/relaxation program that will suit your lifestyle on an ongoing basis.

86+: It is time to start over. At any age you can learn how to adapt more efficiently. You will need a guide, a teacher, or a coach. Exploring your hidden talents will take up to 3 years of systematic effort. You will need to watch your thoughts, since you need to believe that change is possible. Be sure to use a mentor who practices the principles of fitness and well-being and also has a sense of humor. As Wayne Dyer states, "When you can believe it, you can see it." Sample activities for fitness and health promotion include:

1. Work with your physician to identify what activities you are ready to participate in.

2. Use a resource person (i.e., physical or occupational therapist) to evaluate your work-station/home to minimize problems by adapting the dimensions (height of chairs, desk, etc.) to meet your individual requirements.

3. Identify a resource person to assist you in enhancing your overall fitness and well-being.

4. Develop an individual health and fitness plan to carry out 12–20 minutes a day as part of daily living (cardiac/coordination/flexibility).

5. For recreation/relaxation, select one or more activities that you enjoy. It is critical to make a commitment to spend 15–30 minutes at physical activities, two to three times a week. Take some time to develop a recreation/relaxation program that will suit your lifestyle on an ongoing basis.

For further information: Osa Jackson–Wyatt, Ph.D., P.T, Physical Therapy Center, 134 W. University, Suite 302, Rochester, MI 48307, (810) 651–4573, Fax (810) 651–5394.©

Chapter IV
Foundation for Support—
Feet To Stand On

IT'S THE END OF THE WORKING DAY and your feet sometimes burn inside your shoes, or it is uncomfortable to stand on your feet. If you lie down and rest with your shoes off and in one, two, three, five, or seven hours your feet slowly feel better, then the following movement experiments may be useful to you. What are movement experiments?

The experiments involve you beginning to have a conversation with yourself and your body about finding the easiest ways to bring yourself back to Natural Ease™. Natural Ease™ can best be described as that gentle, soft, and relaxed state a happy child assumes when resting comfortably. As adults, the ability to use that Natural Ease™ and to return to it at the end of each day is part of what leads to a more pleasant quality of life. It is not uncommon for adults to find it necessary to get some coaching or reminding on how to let go of tension and return to Natural Ease™. Natural Ease™ involves your body, your mind, and your spirit. The questions that need to be answered are:

1. Are you willing to work with yourself?

2. Are you willing to examine what you do and how you do it?

3. Are you willing to make minor changes that could allow you to have an increase in Natural Ease™ anywhere in your body (for this discussion, in your feet)?

If the answer is yes, then let us begin. As the movement experiments proceed, it is important that you take breaks as needed. This means that any time you find you need to stop, or you have the urge to stroke your foot, or the urge to stretch your leg out, then put your foot down on the floor. It is crucial that you take intermissions as you need them, otherwise Natural Ease™ cannot occur. Your mental attitude needs to be: "I will make time for myself to notice the responses in my body." Note that the urge to stretch or change position needs to be followed when it occurs. It is critical to be willing to notice these natural cues (yawn, urge to stretch) that enhance our ability to relax at rest and in action.

Movement Exploration: Finding a Better Way

NOTE: Begin to read the following description and try the movements suggested only if you have normal feet. If you have had surgery or other problems with your feet, please consult your physician about any precautions for movements and exercise.

This material is meant to be read out loud by a friend as you try to do the described movements. Select a friend or relative with whom you enjoy sharing new things to read to you. As you begin, you are looking for the same feeling you had as a small child when a friend came over to play—the attitude that says, "It's fun trying something new." Begin to actually do the movements with this gentle, playful mindset. Learning to move with greater ease can only happen by "doing," noticing how well the effort worked and then making corrections as needed. You are looking for natural, easy learning, and there is no need to rush or force yourself. If you have no one you wish to share this with, then you can read the material onto an audio tape. Read each sentence at least twice. Speak slowly enough that it is easy to follow the directions and you feel there is enough time to try the suggested movements.

Sit down in a comfortable chair. As you sit in the chair, it is important to notice if you can truly rest and get comfortable in the chair (see Chapter I for review, if needed). The first step is to evaluate how you are sitting. Take time to notice how you are sitting. Are your feet providing equal contact with the floor? At rest, the task is for you to notice how the right side feels compared to the left. You are asked to notice any feelings of heaviness, pressure, pulling, tingling, numbness, or pain. So, begin with your feet and ankles. Do they match in how they feel? Some people can notice how they feel with their eyes open; others find it easier with their eyes shut. Try to notice what you feel one way and then the other, and find out which is easiest for you.

Now notice how your ankles feel and if the right and left match. Move your attention to your calves (the back of your lower leg) and note how you feel. Continue to compare right to left and proceed to note how your knees feel just sitting there. Give yourself time to notice; that is the first step in problem solving to find a better way. It is important to be aware of the obvious—pain is a signal that something needs to be adjusted or changed.

Next move your attention to your thighs and note how they feel on top, on the sides, and on the back. Then move your attention to your hips and your sitting bones. Note any differences between the weight on the right and the left. How does your lower back feel?

If you find any areas that are not comfortable while sitting still at rest, please refer to Chapter III, movement experiment 1, to explore ways to make sitting reasonably comfortable. The goal is to start the movement exploration from a position of comfort. It is important to practice feeling comfortable as you move and to be considerate of yourself. If you have pain, there is no reason to practice "painful" motions—you already know how to create pain. The goal of movement exploration is to find an easier and more comfortable way.

Continue to scan your body to notice how you feel just sitting there. How does your middle back feel at the beltline? Is there the same ease on the right side as on the left? Next move your attention to your upper back and your shoulder blades. Do the right and the left sides feel equally comfortable? How about your shoulders, arms, and hands? Does one arm feel the same as the other? Bring your attention to your chest and neck. How does the right side of your neck feel compared to the left? If you notice any areas of pulling, pressure, burning, or other discomfort, refer to Chapter III, movement experiments 2, 3, and 5, for hints on how to get more comfortable before starting the new movement exploration.

Lastly, notice how your scalp and face feel. Make a note of any areas of discomfort. Use Chapter III, movement experiment 4, to get as comfortable as possible. If the advice on positioning and how to modify the chair does not allow you to sit comfortably, then lie on your back and do the movement exploration from that position. The golden rule for discovering your Natural Ease™ is: *You need to start in a position that feels good enough that you want to go back and do some more.*

The more you are aware of all the different areas of yourself that are not resting at ease, the easier it becomes to improve your level of comfort. If needed, put a pillow behind your back so that there is a slight curve just above to just below your waistband and you feel you are well supported. Your thighs need to be parallel to the floor to allow the muscles of the lower back and thighs to rest, and your legs and feet need to be about hip width apart. Your ankles need to be below your knees—not behind them or in front of them, but straight below—so they can provide good solid support. Breathing needs to be natural and feel adequate.

Presuming that you can sit comfortably, decide which foot you would like to work on first. (Note: If you cannot sit with ease, lie on your back. Bend one knee and place the foot flat for support. Try to cross the other leg over the knee that is bent and rest the ankle on the thigh. If you are lying on your back, please take at least two breaths and rest between each movement experiment.) While sitting, take your foot and place it so that the ankle is resting on the thigh of the other leg. The leg that has the foot resting on the floor should be standing comfortably and the knee should be squarely over the ankle. That means the leg is straight up and down. Now take the shoe and sock off the foot that is resting on the thigh of the other leg. Just rest in that position for a moment. Allow yourself to lightly tap the thigh (while your foot is resting on the other thigh). Now begin to stroke the foot gently. Take a few moments to get accustomed to doing the stroking. (If you are on your back, you can use a wooden cooking spoon with a washcloth wrapped around the end and tied securely to stroke the foot.) Repeat the gentle stroking of every part of the foot, taking frequent rests. (If you are lying down, only do this stroking with the spoon—do not proceed to the next step until you can sit with ease and touch your foot.) As you look at your foot, allow yourself to say—"I have a foot, and I want to learn how to use myself (my foot) more comfortably." Avoid critical statements like "my foot is too big, too broad, too calloused." Simply come to accept that you have a foot, and that your goal at this moment is to experiment to see how your foot can move with greater ease.

Now place the palm of one hand on the sole of your foot and the palm of the other hand on top of your foot. Rest in this position for a moment and notice how you feel. Make any adjustments to get more comfortable. (Place one or two pillows under your head if lying on your back.) Now begin to stroke your palms along your foot so that the last thing that touches your toes is the heel of your hands. Then place your palms near the back of your ankle and slide the flat of your hands (one on top and one on the bottom) forward along your foot to the toes, continuing off the end of your foot. Do the stroking motion gently, as though you are touching the foot of someone you care about. Stroke your foot with an attitude of curiosity (i.e., How does this feel and can I make it easier?). If you find you are resisting, angry, or unable to remain in a supportive state of mind toward yourself, you may want to stop and seek some outside help. It's difficult to learn when you are angry, feeling frustrated, or thinking negative thoughts about yourself. Finding out how to make your body work better by observation and doing small movements and experiments requires the ability to talk to yourself and convince yourself that you are ready to change (letting go of any negative emotions). If you have anger toward yourself or your body, or anger toward someone who you think caused you to have an accident or injury, then it is necessary to seek help from a counselor, minister, rabbi, or a trusted friend so that you can let go of the anger or fear and come to a learning attitude. To learn Natural Ease™ of movement, it is helpful to release feelings of anger over events of the past and live in the present.

If you proceed, it is presumed that your attitude is one of desiring to learn to move with greater ease, balance, and coordination. Check that your ankle is at rest. The way to do that is by taking the hand that is on the same side as the foot that is resting on the floor and just tap the foot that is resting across the thigh of the other leg. The ankle is supposed to be pliable and totally relaxed. How do you know your ankle is relaxed? Move your big toe toward the ceiling and then let go of the effort and drop your foot to the resting position. When your foot is at rest and there is no effort to hold it up, that is the position you need to start from.

Now take the hand that is easiest to reach your toes with (it does not matter which hand) and begin to gently stroke each toe. Start at the baby toe and place one finger on top of the toe and one beneath it and gently stroke your fingers along the length of the toe, past the toenail, and totally let go. Repeat the stroking motion for each toe of your foot, one at a time—slowly, smoothly, and comfortably. Stop and notice your comfort level after stroking each toe. Breathing needs to be natural (avoid holding your breath). When you have stroked all five toes, lift your leg down and put the foot flat on the floor. Check whether there is numbness, tingling, or discomfort, and note if you are sitting reasonably well. If you notice any discomfort or problems, stop and rest. Explore ways to increase your comfort, such as using pillows for support. Continue the movement exploration with your foot only after you have made yourself comfortable.

Taking the same foot, place it across your thigh so that the ankle is resting on the thigh of the opposite leg. You can place a small towel or pillow on your thigh if that makes the contact between the thigh of one leg and the side of the calf/ankle of the other leg more comfortable. Begin to repeat the process of gently inviting each toe to become longer, starting with the smallest toe, stroking the toes as you did earlier. It should be a gentle invitation—not pulling and certainly not making the joint pop. The gentle stroking should cause no pain and no discomfort. Each time you get to the great toe (the biggest toe) return to the baby toe and start the sequence over again. Be sure the rest of you is comfortable. The motion is a gentle sliding of your fingers along the top and bottom of your toe, from the base of the toe out toward the tip, and then moving on to the next toe. Your breathing needs to be relaxed. There should be no major effort in your arms as you gently invite each toe to become longer, and as you finish each toe, proceed to the next one.

Presuming you feel comfortable, begin with the baby toe and gently pull and at the same time roll the toe between your two fingers. Go on to the next toe, gently pulling and rolling that toe between your fingers. The gentle pulling is a traction and an invitation to the toe to become slightly longer. Repeat the slight traction movement and the rolling between your fingers for each toe. As you do this, it is again important to notice: Is the movement pain free? Is the activity comfortable? How do I need to do this to ensure my comfort? *It is important that you not drag or force yourself toward improvement.* It is your job to find the small movement that can invite change. As you listen to the directions, repeat the procedure with each toe. Rest as needed. When you get to the great toe you can start over at the baby toe or stop and rest, whichever feels right for you.

It is assumed that you are gently doing the traction movement to one toe, rolling the toe between your fingers, and proceeding to the next toe. It is presumed that your breathing is not disturbed, meaning that your breathing goes on by itself and is not punctuated or in any way interrupted by the movements of your fingers/toes. As you discover an area that might be uncomfortable or a toe that may be tender, then do less—use a lighter, gentler touch. It is an exploration to learn about yourself. *How do I need to change what I'm doing so I can find the pain-free movement that helps me to learn Natural Ease™?* This is the goal. The pain-free way to learn is using that amount of contact and support with your hand that allows the movement of your toe to occur without discomfort or pressure elsewhere in your foot, leg, or other parts of your body.

At this point, stop and stroke your entire foot again using both palms. Place the palm of one hand on the bottom of your foot and the palm of the other hand on the top. Simultaneously stroke your foot as though it is the foot of someone you care about. Now place your foot flat on the floor and rest. Notice how the foot you have stroked rests on the ground and supports you compared to the foot you have not stroked. Make a mental note of any differences in length, heaviness, comfort, skin color, temperature, or resting position of the toes on the floor.

Presuming you are sitting comfortably and have rested long enough, place the same foot back on your thigh again. If it is not easy at this point to have the same foot on your thigh, you can stop and repeat the activity you just completed using your other foot, prior to going on with new activities. If you are uncomfortable, it is very important to realize that you may need to use even less effort, or you may need to modify your sitting posture to be more comfortable. Prioritize comfort as you explore the movements—do a little less, use more support (pillows, towel), and make changes to allow Natural Ease™.

The last part of the sequence involves taking one hand (the opposite one of the foot you are using) and interlacing the fingers between the toes (palm on the sole of the foot) so that your baby finger goes between the baby (smallest) toe and the one next to it, and so on, so that your thumb is on the outside of your big toe. Sit in this position as long as is easy, or up to 3 minutes as desired. Your ankle should still be relaxed (not pulled up toward the ceiling but just hanging with no effort at all)—a "jello" ankle, meaning there is no effort on your part to stay in that position. Allow your fingers to interlace easily, placing them at the base where the toe is attached to the foot, or if that is not easy, move them down as far as is reasonable for you. If you cannot get all four fingers between your toes, then stop and collect four pencils and place them between your toes instead. Placing your fingers (or the pencils) between your toes provides an invitation for them to change (widen, lengthen, and relax).

Is this movement too much? If you are not feeling at ease, then do less; move your fingers or the pencils up toward the tip of your toes to make the activity easier. Be sure all toes are participating equally. Don't force yourself. *The movement exploration is a game to learn about yourself.* Proceed at a pace so that you enjoy the game and are still curious to learn more. You cannot rush learning to move with greater ease, balance, and coordination. Learning cannot occur, and you certainly won't want to return to the land of new discovery, if it is not a reasonably pleasant experience.

Take your fingers from between your toes and gently stroke your foot as you did before, with the palm of one hand on the sole of the foot and the palm of the other hand on top of the foot at the same time, sliding down the foot so the last thing you touch is your toes. Again, just straighten your leg, put the foot flat on the floor, and sit. Notice the foot you have been stroking: How does the foot look compared to the other one? How does the foot feel compared to the other one? Changes in color, temperature, comfort level, or heaviness may occur—but they may not occur. What is the goal? The goal is to find a comfortable way to come to Natural Ease™ (movement to get the task done with comfort, balance, and a sense of coordination).

The road to Natural Ease™ is not a forced, strenuous road; it involves easy, comfortable activity and observation. If you have gone beyond the level of ease and find you are uncomfortable, stop and start over again tomorrow. It is important to explore what happens when you use a little less effort. At times it is necessary to start with movements that are microscopic in size (so small that if someone looks at you, they can barely see you moving) and get comfortable before you increase to bigger motions.

If you are still doing fine, go ahead and bring your foot up one more time. Using the same leg as before, cross the ankle and let it rest on the thigh of your other leg, Now do the previous movement exploration again, this time using your other hand. Instead of the hand opposite from the leg that is resting on your thigh, use the hand on the same side of your body (right hand for the right foot, left hand for the left foot). Where you previously started from the sole of your foot to interlace the fingers between the toes, this time start from the top of your foot. Once again, make sure your ankle is at rest, and only place the fingers as far between the toes as is comfortable. The position of the fingers is an invitation to change. Ask yourself: Can I soften, can I relax, can I allow a change? A change is a spontaneous improvement using my brain and all my abilities to soften and change how my feet and my entire body are at rest.

Remember, if your fingers feel too thick to do the experiment comfortably, use pencils, and gradually over time change to thicker pencils or pens until you can use your fingers. As you allow your fingers (or pencils) to rest between your toes, an additional exploration you can do is to take the other hand and gently tap your foot four or five times along the arch and the big toe so the foot vibrates—tap, tap, tap and then rest. Repeat the tapping at comfortable intervals. Again, it is presumed that you are comfortable and have no pain. Rest between each time you tap your foot. The rest period should last at least as long it takes you to breathe in and breathe out. The time is important to allow you to observe, to notice, to check—How am I feeling? Is there anything I need to do to get more comfortable? You are responsible for exploring to find a better and easier way to do the activity.

Whenever you feel you've had enough, take your fingers out. How long you leave your fingers between your toes should be based on your own observations. The length of time you leave your fingers between your toes is not important. The key question is: Am I helping myself discover a sense of letting go, or relaxing, or becoming aware of a part of myself that needs to soften? The moment you feel the activity is mildly difficult or challenging, stop, take your fingers out, and again stroke your foot slowly by placing the palm of one hand on the top of your foot and the other palm on the bottom of your foot and allowing your fingers to stroke downward. Uncross your leg and place it back on the floor and notice how the foot and leg feel at rest after doing the movement exploration. Notice how the foot on the side you stroked supports your leg compared to the other foot. Then return to the beginning of this chapter and repeat the entire movement exploration for the other foot.

Learning how to work with the tension that builds up in our bodies after vigorous exercise, athletics, injury, or work-related activities is an important part of maturity. Just as one erases a blackboard each day in order to write new information on it the next day, our human bodies repeatedly become tight with excess tension as we interact and work at a fast pace, become tired, or feel rushed. The extra tension comes to assist us, and for the moment, for a short period of time, it is a natural boost to us in performing an activity. Accumulations of excess tension over days or weeks will make your body rigid and tense and more prone to accidents. For this reason, at the end of each day or at the beginning of a new day, the ability to use movement explorations like those for the foot discussed above allow each person to work with the unnecessary tension or stress that has accumulated in the body. Other references for movement lessons that can enhance walking and/or running are listed at the end of this chapter.[1, 2] Natural Ease™ needs to be felt everywhere in your body.

Now that you have completed the movement exploration to help your feet gain that Natural Ease™, it is important to place the shoes you wish to wear next to each foot. It is critical to note whether *the shape of each shoe matches the shape of the foot*. The premise is that if the shoe is smaller or narrower than the foot, there will be some compression of the foot. As you take a step when walking, the front portion of your foot, just below where the toes attach to the body of the foot, needs to broaden as you roll to push off and move your leg forward. In a shoe that is too narrow, the broadening of your foot cannot occur, and as a result, the pushing off motion is hampered. The body is unique and very adaptable. The result of wearing too tight or too narrow a shoe is that your knees will have to be more vigorous in their movement during walking, and the long-term result will be strain and an increased potential for ankle, knee, hip, and back injury, overuse strain, or chronic pain. It is essential that the shoes you wear match the shape of your feet.

At this point, we need to address the question of fashion. You will notice if you wear a shoe with a heel taller than one and a half inches, it will in fact cause your hips to tighten. Therefore, it is recommended that as you work toward Natural Ease™, and you desire your low back curve to be natural at rest, fashionable shoes need to be described as comfortable shoes. It is critical to avoid shoes that cause unnatural postures.

The work of Dr. Moshe Feldenkrais was the basis for these movement experiments, and his theme was "Awareness Through Movement." As you become aware of what you are doing, you can accomplish what you want.[3] If you decide it is important for you to have happy feet, then the movement exploration described can be the beginning of an adventure in attitude and enjoyment and the possibility of returning to comfortable sitting, standing, and walking. It is presumed that you would do both feet several times per week in the same manner. Judge for yourself how many repetitions and how much time is comfortable. Stop and start as needed so you become acquainted with and get used to the state of Natural Ease™. For many, the Natural Ease™ disappears slowly, and until pain occurs they are unaware that it is gone. Your body can become so tense that you almost feel numb.

Natural Ease™ involves a level of comfort where we can choose to make room for ourselves and our comfort. Take your time and get acquainted. Natural Ease™ is a human necessity! If over the years people have told you hard work is the only honest thing to do, you will need to trust and understand that this idea only applies up to a certain point. The old adage "no pain, no gain" is a military training philosophy that applies to preparing people psychologically and physically for war. As you try to increase your comfort level and movement efficiency and to rediscover Natural Ease™ for any desired activity, all exploration needs to be done so you feel comfortable and have the desire to repeat the movements. That is the level of comfort you are looking for. If you find that this provokes you and makes you feel that it's too easy—too slow—too small—too nice, then perhaps you should stop and talk with a friend, a minister, or a counselor about it. If life has been a struggle for a long time, it can cause increased tightness and tension in the body, and it is not uncommon that you will require some time to get used to the feeling of Natural Ease™. This means you will need to get reacquainted with the wonderful privilege and the ability to stand and walk on your feet without pain or a sense of strain, of feeling comfortable both at rest and during daily activities.

Experiment with these ideas and, if in doubt, do a little smaller movement and use a little less effort. Please feel free to share your reactions, your comments, and your questions in a letter. Address them to Osa Jackson-Wyatt, Ph.D., P.T., Physical Therapy Center, 134 W. University, Suite 302, Rochester, MI 48307 (please send a self-addressed stamped envelope).

References

1. Heggie, J. *Running With The Whole Body.* Emmaus, PA: Rodale Press, 1986.

2. Zemach–Bersin, D.; Zemach–Bersin, K., and Reese, M. *Relaxercise.* New York: Harper Collins, 1990.

3. Feldenkrais, M. *Awareness Through Movement.* New York: Harper & Row, 1979.